Praise for
How to Help the One You Love by
Brad Lamm

"The deeply dedicated counselor presents a four-step method based in his experiences on both sides of the process. . . . As a thorough guide to helping substance abusers find help, this makes a valuable addition to the self-help shelves."

—*Publishers Weekly* (starred review)

"Lamm's step-by-step approach empowers families and friends to change their loved ones through compassionate, caring, and continuing support."

—Mehmet Oz, MD, host of *The Dr. Oz Show*

PENGUIN BOOKS

Quit Vaping

Brad Lamm, CIP, is an interventionist best known for helping people make life-enhancing change on *The Doctors, The Dr. Oz Show, Dr. Phil*, and *Today*. He has managed more than a thousand interventions, visited hundreds of treatment facilities across the globe, presented before Parliament in Britain, served on the board of the Association of Intervention Specialists, collaborated with the most knowledgeable recovery treatment specialists, and worked at the state level to reform treatment options to various communities. He is the author of *How to Help the One You Love* and *Just 10 Lbs.*, and in 2012 he founded Breathe Life Healing Center, which uses industry-leading techniques to provide powerful rehabilitation for body, mind, and spirit. He lives with his family in Los Angeles, California.

Quit Vaping

YOUR FOUR-STEP,
28-DAY PROGRAM TO
STOP SMOKING
E-CIGARETTES

Brad Lamm, CIP

Foreword by Mehmet Oz, MD

life

PENGUIN BOOKS
An imprint of Penguin Random House LLC
penguinrandomhouse.com

ISBN 9780143135876 (paperback)
ISBN 9780525507451 (ebook)

Printed in the United States of America
1 3 5 7 9 10 8 6 4 2

Set in Iowan Old Style
Designed by Chris Welch

Our doubts are traitors,
And make us lose the good we oft might win
By fearing to attempt.

—William Shakespeare,
Measure for Measure, act 1, scene 4

Contents

Part Three: Your Quit Kit

Foreword

When I was five years old, 42 percent of American adults were addicted to nicotine. It was a form of the all-American normal. Doctors even appeared in advertisements promoting the healthful qualities of cigarettes and smoking.

By 1980, when I was in college, 33 percent smoked. Health-care experts were waking up to the impact of smoking on the body and the power of nicotine as a drug. Still, in the 1980s, cigarettes were Hollywood cool; glossy magazine pages made smoking hip. We were beginning to understand the dangers and long-term health costs, but back then it was still cool.

As views on nicotine addiction changed, as I was stepping from medical school into the operating theater, I had to ask myself how I would approach it in my own life and practice. I loved helping hearts get better and gave it 110 percent every time I worked on such a precious part, the one that is everybody's engine, and a part of the human body so terribly impacted by smoking. So what to do? An answer soon became clear: I would address it head-on. I decided not to operate on patients who continued to smoke cigarettes. I would stand up and promise to give my all if they gave their all and quit. I became a smoking interventionist, as it were, sitting down with patients and saying, "Hey, I really want to help you and work on your heart, but to do that I need you to stop smoking. I want you to live as long and as healthily as possible." Through my show and the work I do, I have touched millions of hearts, lungs, and lives. Today only 18 percent of Americans smoke, and this book will help more people trade nicotine for breathing easier.

Understand that nicotine is one of the most addictive drugs on the planet—and the one that affects more individuals than any other—bar none. Addiction is driving this epidemic! We are racing to respond in real time to today's vaping public health crisis. Headlines tick up the death count, and stories describe how our young sons and daughters are developing profoundly diseased lungs from vaping, even as we grapple with helping more than 10 million addicted Americans.

This new book combines the best science and theory to help people give up the nicotine itch. I encourage you to start this simple program and let Brad or the ones you love help you quit vaping for good. Brad and I have known each other a long time, and we have worked together to interrupt families in crisis, to help them say YES to a better life. Today, as you hold this book, we ask you in unison to quit for good. This is my invitation to you as a doctor: Be courageous. Honor your heart, head, and body as well as those you love.

Commit to the next four weeks, and I believe this book will help you quit for good. You are not alone, and as Brad says, together we can do more than we can do apart.

—Mehmet Oz, MD

Introduction

Anew epidemic is killing people.

In America, the first death attributed to vaping occurred on August 23, 2019, in Illinois. The state's department of public health announced the sad news, but in order to protect the person's privacy, officials didn't release the person's name, age, gender, or exact location. Since then, forty more people have died from vaping-related illness. The youngest was just thirteen years old, which underscores the devastating effects that e-cigarettes are having on teenagers. In fact, most victims of vaping-related illness are younger than thirty-five.

The media reports alarming stories, almost daily, about the vaping crisis. Damage to vapers' lungs has become so prevalent that the Centers for Disease Control and Prevention (CDC) has coined a new acronym for it: EVALI, or e-cigarette, vaping-associated lung injury. Instances of EVALI are surging. As of February 2020, the CDC has confirmed more than 2,700 cases of vaping-related lung injury in addition to the reported deaths.

After several days of high fever and flulike symptoms, people suffering from EVALI rush into emergency rooms with shortness of breath and difficulty breathing. One twenty-one-year-old man in Utah had such severe lung damage from vaping that even a ventilator couldn't help him breathe. Doctors had to connect him to a machine that pumped oxygen directly into his bloodstream to keep him alive. Closer examination of his lung fluid revealed that fat had clogged his white blood cells—not from the chemicals that he had vaped, but likely from the breakdown of his own lung tissue. Doctors thought that he might die, but thankfully he survived and, after a two-week stay in the hospital, went home.

Vapers are dying, and their lungs are failing, but medical officials still don't know what lasting damage and other health problems vaping will cause in the long run.

So how did we get here?

Smoking Tobacco

It all starts with tobacco, a plant that contains large amounts of the nicotine chemical. The native people of Mesoamerica and South America discovered tobacco and the physical results of smoking its dried leaves, and Native Americans throughout the New World often used it in medical and ceremonial contexts. Europeans learned of it from them in the early 1500s and, from there, gradually introduced it to the rest of the world.

In 1559, Jean Nicot—the Frenchman from whose name the word *nicotine* derives—introduced tobacco to France, and a dozen or so years later English explorers introduced it to their own homeland. Walter Raleigh brought samples from Virginia's Roanoke Colony to the court of Queen Elizabeth I, but not everyone believed in this captivating new plant. In 1604, just one year into his reign, King James I of England called smoking tobacco "a custom loathsome to the eye, hateful to the nose, harmful to the brain, dangerous to the lungs, and in the black, stinking fume thereof, nearest resembling the horrible Stygian smoke of the pit that is bottomless."

Despite those protestations, the burgeoning tobacco trade helped the English support Jamestown, their first permanent settlement in the New World. In 1612, John Rolfe became the first European settler in North America to grow tobacco as a cash crop, and the plant soon became known as the "golden weed." King James I wasn't the only person who recognized the dangers of smoking this enticing new plant, however. Shortly thereafter, a sultan of the Ottoman Empire and an emperor of China both issued edicts banning smoking it. Powerful leaders knew centuries before the rise of modern medicine that smoking tobacco posed a major health risk to their people.

Lung cancer deaths related to smoking increased sharply in 1965 and continued through the 1990s. What was once touted as safe by doctors was killing untold numbers. The backlash against cigarette makers resulted in the Master Settlement Agreement of November 1998, brokered between the four largest tobacco companies in America and the attorneys general of forty-six states. Its stipulations included that those companies had to curb or cease certain advertising practices as well as to pay the states *forever* to compensate them for the medical costs of people with smoking-related illnesses. The settlement money also funded an antismoking advocacy group called Truth Initiative.

Even after all that medical proof and toxic publicity,

smoking cigarettes still kills nearly half a million people every year just in America, according to the CDC. That's almost one in five deaths. Smoking also strongly increases your odds of developing many life-threatening diseases, including chronic obstructive pulmonary disease (COPD), lung cancer, other cancers, heart disease, and stroke.

The Rise of Vaping

When e-cigarettes first hit the market in 2007, it seemed as though we had found a high-tech solution to the world's toughest-to-break habit. As a form of harm reduction, vaping was supposed to help chronic smokers quit and thus avoid the cancer-causing tar in cigarettes. It even looked cool. Some devices resembled flash drives and required charging like other fun pieces of tech.

You'll hear that vaping is safer than smoking, but it's not. Vaping is just a different form of smoking, and the latest scientific research shows that e-cigarettes are just as bad as traditional cigarettes—maybe worse. Smoking kills people slowly, over many years. As we've seen, vaping can kill quickly, within months or a year.

EVALI can strike anyone, but it's disproportionately affecting males, who make up 70 percent of all cases. Right now, an estimated 15 million American adults use e-cigarettes. The oldest patient to fall ill was seventy-five, and two people over fifty recently died in Minnesota. According to the CDC, e-cigs are the most commonly used smoking product among teens, and roughly 4 million teens have become vapers. Between 2017 and 2018, vaping increased among teenagers by a shocking 78 percent. That trend will continue unless officials take serious action.

Because of the surge in teen vaping, the FDA "plans" on curbing e-cigarette sales, but they haven't yet. You'll learn more about why that hasn't happened in "Myths and Truths." CDC officials are notifying health-care systems and clinics across the country about vaping-related illnesses. State health departments are issuing dire warnings. At least one major manufacturer has stopped making fruit-flavored products. That's a decent start, but none of that's enough. That's also not why you're reading this book. You're reading it because either you want to quit vaping or you know someone who wants to quit.

Before we dive into the mechanics of how to do that, let's take a closer look at nicotine and vaping.

Nicotine

Tobacco belongs to the nightshade family of plants, which, on the nutritional side, includes bell peppers, cayenne pepper, eggplant, paprika, and tomatoes. The family also includes belladonna, a lethal poison, and farmers once used nicotine as an insecticide. Nicotine is an alkaloid stimulant that occurs in high concentrations in tobacco leaves. It's toxic and highly addictive. The CDC cautions that nicotine dependence is the most common form of addiction in America and that nicotine is as addictive as heroin, cocaine, and alcohol. Nicotine also functions as a gateway drug because it lowers the addiction threshold for other drugs, including cocaine, methamphetamines, and opioids.

E-cigarette producers process the nicotine from tobacco leaves into vaping liquid, and their products can get nicotine into your system as fast as a cigarette. Case in point: one popular e-cig brand brags that its vaping device has a nicotine content equal to that of regular cigarettes and that it gets that nicotine into your system more than 2.5 times faster than competing brands. Some people can blow through one vaping pod or cartridge in just a few hours, which is a huge amount of nicotine to absorb that quickly!

The nicotine in some vapes also goes down more easily than regular cigarettes. The vape juice in one brand, for example, contains nicotine salts. Unlike regular cigarettes, which can hurt the throat and lungs, nicotine salts don't cause the same irritation. According to an opinion piece in *The New England Journal of Medicine*, this "advance" in nicotine chemistry may make vaping even more addictive.

Nicotine also accelerates your heart rate, raises your blood pressure, and elevates your blood sugar levels. As we'll see, it can damage the brains and lungs of young people in particular. In large enough doses, it can cause nicotine poisoning, which can kill.

The Chemistry of Nicotine in the Body

Regardless of how nicotine enters your body, it travels through your bloodstream to your brain, where nicotine levels peak in about ten seconds. This "hit" dissipates just as quickly, along with its associated feelings of reward, such as relaxation. Even though the chemical is a stimulant, smoking it feels relaxing because it temporarily alleviates the addiction, which causes a surge of feel-good endorphins. But this surge lasts for a much shorter time than with other drugs, which is why you feel the need to smoke or vape so often: to maintain the drug's pleasurable effects.

As you continue to use nicotine, your body craves more and more of it to feel the same as it did when you used less. That feedback loop causes the addiction and makes it harder to quit. Over time, nicotine can change the way your brain works and interfere with the normal function of your brain chemicals. For many people, long-term brain changes can affect their ability to learn, manage stress, and exercise self-control. At that point, they need to use nicotine regularly just to maintain normal brain function.

More Than Just Nicotine

In addition to nicotine, vape juice, when heated, produces an aerosol that may contain dozens of chemicals. They include: benzene, formaldehyde, and propylene glycol, which is an ingredient in antifreeze. It also contains diacetyl, a chemical linked to "popcorn lung," another debilitating, potentially fatal lung disease.

The vape market features more than 450 different brands of e-cigarettes and nearly 8,000 flavored liquids, with hundreds more appearing each month. Mango certainly sounds tastier than menthol, and it might seem safe and delicious—but it's not. Inhaling flavors is worse than eating them because our digestive systems are better than our lungs at absorbing liquids. Even the Flavor and Extract Manufacturers Association, a not-for-profit organization that works with government officials to ensure the safety of flavoring substances, says, "It is false and misleading to claim that food-grade flavorings are safe to vape."

As many media stories have reported, manufacturers create flavors specifically to target young vapers. Are we seriously supposed to believe that flavors such as bubble gum or cotton candy are helping *adults* make the switch from smoking cigarettes? If those flavors don't sound so bad, other youth-targeted flavors include cinnamon roll, peanut butter cup, and riffs on pretty much every sugary cereal in the breakfast aisle of a grocery store.

Vaping THC

THC stands for tetrahydrocannabinol, and it's the main psychoactive ingredient in marijuana. Various countries and states have decriminalized and legalized marijuana, and the House Judiciary Committee recently approved a bill legalizing it on the federal level in America. As the criminal and social stigma dissipates, more people are vaping marijuana with THC cartridges purchased from dealers online or on the street.

An editorial published in *The New England Journal of Medicine* concluded that the majority of—but not all—people affected by EVALI used vapes containing THC. According to the CDC, the offending chemical in these cases is vitamin E acetate, a petroleum-derived oil used in cosmetics and topical medications. It's safe when consumed in foods or used on the skin, but scientists say that when inhaled it has adverse effects on the lungs. In tests of lung fluids from people with EVALI, CDC researchers found traces of vitamin E acetate in twenty-nine samples from ten different states. Two of the patients had died.

Vitamin E acetate appeared on the illicit THC market in spring 2019 as a thickening and cutting agent for THC cartridges. When heated and inhaled through a vape, the chemical returns to an oil form when it reaches the lungs. That oil is enormously sticky, and it coats the lungs like honey, causing major damage.

Teens are vaping marijuana in a variety of ways. They can vape the pulverized leaves or buds themselves, a waxy substance called dabs, or THC and CBD oils. (CBD stands for cannabidiol, a chemical also found in the marijuana plant. It has no psychoactive properties, but it does act as an anti-inflammatory.) As the market for pot becomes legal and expands, many companies are manufacturing devices to vape it from the plant, dabs, or oils, creating a booming but still unregulated industry.

My Mission

Few people seem to know how to help vapers, particularly teenagers, quit. A 2018 *New York Times* article said as much in its headline: "ADDICTED TO VAPED NICOTINE, TEENAGERS HAVE NO CLEAR PATH TO QUITTING." A recent CNBC documentary on vaping drew a similar conclusion: "No one knows how to help you stop."

To date, most addiction specialists have relied on techniques used to help smokers quit, but it's not the same thing. For starters, vapers don't identify themselves as smokers, so all the campaigns and programs directed at smokers aren't reaching vapers in the same way. The social stigmas are different. Vapers skew demographically younger. FDA regulations are lacking, as is manufacturer quality control, and producers are confusing vapers intentionally with mixed messages about health and safety risks.

All of that is why I decided to write this book. It extends a personal mission that has led me across the country, around the world, and into a career that I never envisioned for myself. Earlier in my life, I worked as a successful weather anchor at a top ten TV morning show. But by night multiple addictions ruled my life: food, alcohol, cigarettes, and crystal methamphetamine. At one point, tiny blood vessels were bursting all over my face, and my hands developed a tremor. It felt like I was dying. I was just thirty-five years old.

In a rare moment of lucidity, terrifying realities hit me: *How long will it take before I drive home wasted and kill someone? How long can I keep living like this? Do I want to die like this?*

Soon after, I checked into a rehabilitation center, which began a brutal journey from hopelessness to healing. I got sober in rehab, and since then I have remained in recovery without relapse. From that point, I dedicated my life to helping addicts of all types recover for good and get their lives back on track and to helping families get their loved ones into treatment.

Of my four addictions, nicotine was absolutely the toughest to break. Cigarettes felt like my best friend—*who wanted to kill me*. When I realized that I wasn't giving something up but was taking back control of my life, I found the strength that I needed in order to quit. For other people, as I've seen, it's not that easy.

Throughout my recovery journey, I studied nicotine addiction, learned how cigarettes keep smokers hooked, identified the cues perpetuating the habit, and researched the disastrous health consequences. Since changing the trajectory of my life, I have worked with many people who have struggled with all types of addictions to change the course of their lives. In my work as an interventionist and teacher, I have helped whole families recover from the effects of one individual's addiction. As a result, I recognized the need for a science-based detox program to help people quit.

The Program

My unique, groundbreaking solution to help e-cigarette users, including teens, kick the habit comes from a four-step vaping intervention used at my Breathe Life Healing Centers, a leading residential facility for treating addiction, eating disorders, and trauma. The first of its kind to present a comprehensive solution to quit vaping, the program uses a twenty-first-century approach that's evidence based, results oriented, and has a high rate of success.

As you've seen from the contents, the book consists of three parts. Part One debunks the pervasive myths and lies about vaping and replaces them with truth and facts. It delves deeper into the details about how the body becomes addicted to nicotine, and, if you're the parent or guardian of a teen vaper, it provides no-nonsense guidance on helping your kid quit.

Part Two consists of the four-step quit program. Step One shows you how to plan your quit. Step Two gives you techniques to help you manage your cravings. Step Three helps you reprogram your life, and Step Four gets you across the finish line.

In Part Three, you'll find your Quit Kit. In it, you'll complete the daily assignments of the program and develop personalized means to help you break your habit. This strategic journal and tool kit will help you reinforce your resolve, provide reassurance when you're struggling, and, when you read back through it, give you positive perspective on how far you've come. Use it every day of the program and refer to it after you've finished.

Attention: Parents

This program works for teens! Carefully read the Teen Talk sidebars throughout the book. They speak directly to you about issues that you're facing as the parent or guardian of a teen vaper, and they offer real-world, battle-tested solutions.

The program works for vapers of any age and gives you simple, specific steps to take day by day. Among other actions, you will learn how to create a quit plan, build a support team, follow a nicotine detox, change your inner dialogue, manage your cravings, avoid your triggers, celebrate your achievements, and become a nonvaper. Along the way, lots of exercises, hacks, strategies, and success stories will help you get there.

The book also includes an appendix on how to intervene with vaping friends or family, showing you how to encourage them lovingly and effectively to stop vaping for good.

Recovering from a nicotine addiction is a process of gradual release from one of the world's most addictive drugs. *Quit Vaping* provides the framework for making that happen. I've used my program successfully with thousands of people who wanted to reclaim vibrant, healthy lives, and through this book I want it to reach many more. With a determination to quit and a willingness to do the work, it takes just four steps and twenty-eight short days to quit—just like that.

Quit
Vaping

Part One

Lies and Facts

MYTHS AND TRUTHS

n May 2018, a thirty-eight-year-old man was vaping at his home in St. Petersburg, Florida, when the device's battery exploded. Metal fragments from his vape pen shot into his skull, killing him instantly and igniting a fire at the same time, according to the St. Petersburg deputy fire marshal, as quoted in a CNBC article on the deadly event. It was the first vaping accident fatality in America.

Officials attributed the malfunction to a drop-in battery called the 18650. Certain types of e-cigs called mechanical mods, which allow vapers to control the intensity of their vaping experiences, use this battery. Vapers have to remove the 18650s and recharge them regularly. Repeatedly removing this battery from and reinserting it into vaping devices or chargers can damage its insulating wrapper, compromising the safety of the battery and increasing the risk of explosion. If a vaper draws too much power off the 18650 or if it's damaged, metal-on-metal contact can cause it to explode.

Because it allows users to throttle the power level, the 18650 has grown popular among hard-core vapers, and despite the risk of death, a robust secondary market for it exists online, particularly on auction sites. As with many products like this sold in secondary forums, you don't know exactly what you're buying. The batteries could be counterfeit or refurbished and fail.

Nor did the St. Petersburg death represent a one-in-a-billion freak occurrence. Similar tragic outcomes have befallen other vapers. In January 2019, the e-cig of a Texas man exploded, shooting a shard of metal into his neck, severing an artery, and killing him, too. He was just twenty-four years old. His name was William Eric Brown.

Calamities like this and the shock and grief they bring continue to dominate headlines. Truth Initiative, America's largest not-for-profit organization dedicated to eradicating tobacco use, has been tracking vaping injuries reported by hospitals and burn centers. "Defective, poorly manufactured, and improperly modified e-cigarettes have been known to explode and cause injury," the organization confirmed. A George Mason University study estimated that between 2015 and 2017 more than two thousand Americans visited emergency rooms to seek treatment for burns from e-cigarettes and injuries related to exploding vaping devices.

If the device itself doesn't kill you, the liquid in it will. But numerous multimillion-dollar companies have a vested interest in convincing everyone that their products are safe and worth buying. That brazen hoax succeeds by means of a diabolically executed marketing and advertising campaign based on smoke and mirrors.

Behind the Smoke Screen

Vaping initially surged in popularity because most people thought that it represented a safer alternative to smoking cigarettes. That belief is categorically false. Vape companies, Big Tobacco, which owns a stake in them, their "research" lackeys, and lobbying groups such as the American Vaping Association have propagated a smoky cloud of myths to obscure the truth about e-cigarettes. Together, they sing a devil's chorus that e-cigs are safe and there's no cause for alarm.

Let's go behind their smoke screen to discover the truth for ourselves. Here are seven dangerous myths about vaping and the corresponding truths that you should know about them.

Myth 1: Vaping can help you quit smoking.

Truth: It won't.

According to the Center on Addiction, a national not-for-profit organization dedicated to stopping substance abuse: "There is little evidence that they [e-cigs] reliably reduce cigarette smoking or lead to smoking cessation. In fact, the nicotine contained in e-cigarettes and other vaping products may actually perpetuate addiction, in some cases making it even harder to quit smoking."

Addiction is addiction. Replacing one harmful addiction with another doesn't make either of them less toxic or either substance less addictive. Harm reduction techniques work best for addictions when based on rigorous scientific evidence and not Big Vape lies. Vaping produces exactly the same cycle of behavior as any other addictive substance: use, response, crave, repeat.

Almost one in twenty American adults uses e-cigarettes, and nearly 60 percent of smokers vape as well. Absorbing two different sets of toxins, more or less simultaneously, can do extreme harm to your body.

Myth 2: Vaping is safer than smoking cigarettes.

Truth: Vaping is as toxic as cigarettes, if not more so.

E-cigarette manufacturers have been feeding people this lie from day one. Smokers burn dried, shredded tobacco leaves and inhale the resulting smoke. Vapers heat a nicotine-based liquid full of noxious chemicals, which produces an inhalable aerosol, commonly called a vapor. One of those toxic chemicals, propylene glycol, dangerously inflames lung tissue.

The media has reported seemingly countless cases of vapers becoming seriously sick or dying, but vape companies still hawk their wares as a safer way to smoke. Many people don't understand, though, that pro-tobacco researchers or scientists paid by Big Tobacco conducted much of the "research" on vaping that has taken place over the last dozen years. That's a blatant, shameful, unscientific conflict of interest.

Because of the alarming increase in instances of EVALI, proper research is heating up. A 2017 study published in the *American Journal of Physiology—Lung Cellular and Molecular Physiology* noted that a rapidly growing body of evidence taken from human studies shows that e-cigarette use has significant lung toxicity, as seen in increasing instances of coughing and phlegm production, bronchitis, asthma, and the frequency and severity of acute bacterial and viral infections.

Vape supporters claim that the risks are relatively unknown, which is also a total lie. Numerous national news outlets reported in August 2019 that medical officials admitted a Utah teen to the ICU who had become so sick from vaping that they had to put her in a medically induced coma in order to treat her. Chest X-rays revealed that she had fat clumps in her lungs linked to the glycerin in the vape juice she had been smoking. Her doctors said that her chest X-rays were some of the worst that they had seen, *ever*.

It doesn't get any clearer than this: according to the CDC, "Besides nicotine, e-cigarettes contain harmful and potentially harmful ingredients, including ultrafine particles that can be inhaled deep into the lungs, flavorants such as diacetyl (a chemical linked to serious lung disease), volatile organic compounds, and heavy metals, such as nickel, tin, and lead."

Myth 3: Vaping products are FDA approved.

Truth: Neither the FDA nor other government agencies have approved or meaningfully regulated vaping products.

The FDA hasn't endorsed e-cigs of any kind for any reason—not even to help people quit smoking—nor has it set any limits on how much nicotine or what other chemicals these devices can contain.

Surprising, right?

From the beginning, officials from the Obama administration who were in the pocket of Big Tobacco either delayed or weakened the regulation of vaping products, setting a precedent for federal inaction. Scott Gottlieb, a physician, once served on the board of a chain of vaping lounges, and President Trump appointed him head of the FDA in 2017. Gottlieb left the agency two years later. Since then, the Trump administration announced that it would ban flavored e-cigarettes, but backlash from the vaping industry prompted officials to reconsider the ban.

Bottom line: a lack of proper governmental regulations allowed an unscrupulous industry to hook a new generation on nicotine.

According to its own website, however, the FDA has taken the following actions:

- All tobacco products, including e-cigarettes, must feature a large, clearly readable warning label: "WARNING: This product contains nicotine. Nicotine is an addictive chemical."
- In August 2016, the FDA made it illegal to sell e-cigarettes and any other kind of electronic nicotine device to people under age eighteen. Retailers are legally responsible for checking photo IDs of anyone under age twenty-seven who tries to buy tobacco products, including e-cigs. As of December 2019, Congress raised the age to twenty-one for nicotine products.
- In July 2019, the FDA announced the launch of its first vape-prevention TV ads educating kids about the dangers of e-cigarette use. The FDA will provide new posters for high schools and educational materials for middle schools across the country.
- The FDA conducts regular inspections of e-cigarette manufacturing facilities, including vape shops that make or modify vaping products. Since 2016, it has conducted more than twelve hundred inspections to confirm that these manufacturers and retailers are complying with regulations, including not selling tobacco products to minors.

But federal regulations still fall short in the marketing and advertising arena. E-cigarette manufacturers can create and spread marketing materials that imply vaping is safe and risk free and that promote the vaping lifestyle as fun and exciting—all of which appeals directly to young adults, teens, and kids.

Myth 4: Vaping has no health risks.

Truth: Vaping can kill you.

Many pro-vaping sources claim that e-cigarettes contain none of the dangers of traditional cigarettes. Again, not true. Drawn from science-based, nonbiased research published in 2018 in the *Annals of the New York Academy of Sciences* and various news reports, here's just a partial list of the terrifying health risks.

Free Radicals: These renegade molecules damage organs and other tissues in your body. They also cause harmful chemical reactions that injure cells, making it difficult for you to resist infections. Vaping juice increases free-radical production and decreases glutathione, a protective free-radical fighter, or antioxidant. Other antioxidants can't function properly without glutathione, which recharges and recycles them. When levels of glutathione drop, your body can't protect its own immune system or detoxify itself.

Weakened Immunity: E-cigarettes can cripple your body's ability to fight unwanted bacteria and weaken the infection-fighting white blood cells that help against viruses, parasites, and fungi. In a 2016 study published in the *American Journal of Physiology—Lung Cellular and Molecular Physiology*, researchers at the University of North Carolina at Chapel Hill analyzed cells scraped from the nasal cavities of volunteers. Some samples came from smokers, some from vapers, and other volunteers did neither. The researchers measured the activity of 594 immunity-linked genes in these cells. In the smoker samples, 53 genes had lower activity levels than usual. Among vapers, those same 53 genes also had lower activity levels, as did another 305 genes. What does that mean? For your immune system, vaping is *worse* for you than smoking.

Lung Damage: In October 2019, pathologists from the Mayo Clinic, America's number one hospital, reviewed the chest X-rays and samples of lung tissue from seventeen people hospitalized after vaping nicotine or marijuana products. The ages of the patients ranged from nineteen to sixty-seven. Two specimens came from people who had died. All of the X-rays showed a pattern of opaque white spots and the appearance of what doctors are calling ground-glass lung.

"All 17 of our cases show a pattern of injury in the lung that looks like a toxic chemical exposure, toxic chemical fume exposure, or a chemical burn injury," said Dr. Brandon Larsen, a surgical pathologist at the Mayo Clinic in Scottsdale, Arizona, as reported in a *New York Times* article. "They look like the kind of change you would expect to see in an unfortunate worker in an industrial accident where a big barrel of toxic chemicals spills and that person is exposed to toxic fumes and there is a chemical burn in the airways."

He added that the damage resembled exposure to the chemical weapons used in World War I. *The New England Journal of Medicine* published the Mayo Clinic team's findings in October 2019.

A study published in *Cancer Prevention Research* in October 2019 reported the first evidence of lung inflammation directly correlated with e-cig use. The study involved nonsmoking volunteers who, for research purposes, used e-cigarettes twice a day for one month. The e-cigs contained no nicotine or flavoring, but they did contain propylene glycol and glycerin, as many vape juices do, which the medical researchers linked to increases in inflammatory cell counts in participants' lungs. The study results suggest that even short-term vaping can cause measurable damage at the cellular level. We know that respiratory inflammation from nicotine exposure can drive lung cancer and other diseases, such as incurable COPD, so vaping does double damage to the lungs.

These problems aren't theoretical or happening in the distant future, either. They're happening *now*. In July 2019, Children's Hospital of Wisconsin admitted eight teenagers with severe lung damage that doctors suspected stemmed from vaping. Their acute symptoms included extreme coughing, shortness of breath, and relentless fatigue. Some had lost significant amounts of weight from vomiting and diarrhea. Dr. Louella Amos, a pediatric pulmonologist who treated the teens, told the *Milwaukee Journal Sentinel* that the kids had reached "the point where they can't breathe." She noted that the symptoms developed rapidly and didn't result from consistent use over time.

Serious lung damage doesn't always result from the vitamin E acetate in THC vapes, either. Jeremy, a twenty-nine-year-old medical technician, worked at a small hospital owned by Breathe Life Healing Centers. The vape juice he used didn't contain vitamin E acetate or THC but rather a vegetable oil, which, when heated, can prove just as harmful. In 2019, medical officials had to put him into a medical coma to treat the damage to his lungs from inhaling that oil. Jeremy survived—just barely—and later asked me to help him quit vaping. All vapes contain oil, and the harm it causes when inhaled is unlike anything that many medical experts have seen before.

Liver Damage: E-cigarette aerosol contains propylene glycol. Your liver metabolizes that chemical into propionaldehyde, which is related to formaldehyde, a known carcinogen as classified by the National Cancer Institute. When propionaldehyde accumulates in the body, it increases the potential for severe liver damage.

Vision Damage: According to a 2015 study in *Current Eye Research*, nicotine decreases the thickness of the retina, which can jeopardize your vision. The other chemicals in e-cigs can accumulate in the retina as well, so vapers run the risk of double damage to their eyes and even blindness.

Heart Problems: West Virginia University studies with lab animals show that vaping can stiffen arteries, leading to cardiovascular injury. In other animal studies, vaping aerosol caused reduced heart function, pericardial edema (a dangerous buildup of fluid around the heart), and even heart malformation. A recent study by researchers at the University of California, San Francisco, concluded that daily use of e-cigarettes may double your odds of a heart attack.

Cancer: Scientists are investigating whether e-cigarettes cause cancer in animals and humans. Vaping aerosol contains cancer-causing chemicals, such as propionaldehyde, as well as trace metals such as aluminum, cadmium, nickel, and tin. A 2019 review published in *Biological Trace Element Research* associates those metals in particular with lung, mouth, and nasal cancers.

A 2018 study published in the *Proceedings of the National Academy of Sciences* found that e-cig vapor caused DNA damage in the lungs and bladders of mice and inhibited DNA repair in their lung tissue. Of forty mice exposed to e-cigarette vapor containing nicotine over the course of fifty-four weeks, 22 percent developed lung cancer, and 57 percent developed precancerous lesions in their bladders.

As for humans, a study by the University of Southern California, published in the *International Journal of Molecular Sciences* in 2019, found that vapers develop some of the same molecular changes in oral tissue that cause cancer in cigarette smokers.

Fetal Development Problems: Nicotine easily passes through the placenta and can accumulate in a fetus's bloodstream in concentrations higher than in the mother's blood. Medical researchers have shown that in-utero exposure to nicotine likely causes medical and behavioral problems in kids whose mothers smoked during pregnancy. These problems include impaired thinking, hyperactivity, anxiety, asthma, greater addiction potential to nicotine and other drugs, and other disorders. Some vapes deliver more nicotine than regular smokes, so expecting mothers who start vaping in order to stop smoking might cause even *more* harm to their unborn children.

Poisoning: The American Association of Poison Control Centers reports that since 2011 poison control centers have been concerned most about exposures to e-cigarette products and liquid nicotine. Liquid nicotine products contain higher concentrations of the chemical than most other tobacco products, which increases the risks of nicotine poisoning.

The lethal dose of nicotine is a moving target scientifically because toxicity depends on a person's age, gender, size, tolerance to the chemical, and other factors. Some studies estimate that 50 to 60 milligrams can kill an adult who weighs 150 pounds, while just 10 milligrams will kill a child.

One cigarette contains about 10 milligrams of nicotine, but smokers absorb only a small amount of the chemical from each cigarette they smoke, around 1 milligram, so you'd have to smoke a *lot* of cigarettes in a very short time to develop nicotine poisoning. As we've seen, the nicotine levels in vape juice, which remains unregulated, vary dramatically. Some contain none, and others may contain 50 milligrams per liter or more.

Mild nicotine poisoning can cause dizziness, tremors, nausea, and vomiting, but more severe cases can lead to life-threatening seizures, slowing of the heart, and even paralysis—particularly in children with a sensitivity to the chemical. Officials need to treat nicotine poisoning fast, otherwise death can occur within an hour. Treatment consists of multiple doses of activated charcoal, which binds to the nicotine molecules and allows the body to expel them. Patients also usually require mechanical ventilation in order to restore their oxygen levels.

Myth 5: All vaping products are the same.

Truth: Vape juices feature a huge range of flavorings and concentrations of nicotine, chemicals, and other toxins.

As we've seen, fewer regulations apply to vaping products than to cigarettes, so they're all a little different. One vape liquid might contain more nicotine than another. The same flavor from two different manufacturers can contain totally different ingredients.

Some producers engineer vape pods or cartridges to deliver a quick, powerful burst of nicotine by adding benzoic acid. It feels more intense, more like a regular cigarette, and as a result that extra chemical makes the liquid even more addictive.

In October 2019, *The New York Times* reported that a former executive of a major vaping company alleged that the company sold at least 1 million contaminated mint-flavored and expired pods and refused to recall them when informed about the problem. It remains unclear how the pods were tainted and with what, but no laws require producers to create quality or even consistent products from batch to batch.

Myth 6: Vaping will keep you from doing other drugs.

Truth: Vaping can act as a gateway to other drugs.

Some people think that if they vape they won't face the temptation to do other drugs or even smoke cigarettes. That just isn't true. Vape devices and cigarettes contain the same addictive toxin: nicotine. Using one won't prevent you from using the other. On the contrary, it might make the transition between them that much easier.

Because the newness of the tech is preserving the cool factor around vaping, the use of e-cigs may be renormalizing smoking behavior. A 2017 study published in *The American Journal of Medicine* revealed that, after eighteen months of vaping, previous nonsmokers are *four* times more likely to start smoking cigarettes. Other studies have revealed that if e-cigarettes didn't come in kid-friendly flavors, young people say they wouldn't vape at all.

Another study, published in *JAMA Pediatrics* in 2017,

suggested that teens who vape are more inclined to take up cigarettes than those who don't. It also observed that kids who switched from e-cigs to cigarettes probably wouldn't have started smoking otherwise.

Vaping can encourage people to try to use other nicotine products, but it doesn't end there. Nicotine itself lowers the body's addiction threshold for other drugs, such as opioids, and stimulants in particular, which include methamphetamines and cocaine.

Myth 7: Exposure to secondhand vape smoke has no health consequences.

Truth: Vape smoke is still dangerous even after being exhaled.

Research has revealed that the aerosol exhaled from e-cigs may contain nicotine and other chemicals. In a 2019 study reported in the *International Journal of Environmental Research and Public Health*, a Dutch research team investigated the potential effects of secondhand vape aerosol on bystanders. The researchers collected the exhaled breath of seventeen volunteers while they were vaping and then analyzed the levels of formaldehyde, glycerol, heavy metals, nicotine, propylene glycol, tobacco-specific nitrosamines (TSNAs, carcinogens created when processing tobacco leaves), and other toxins. The researchers found high levels of copper, nicotine, and propylene glycol in the collected samples.

From these measurements, the researchers estimated bystander exposure for two different scenarios: (1) a nonventilated car with two e-cigarette users and (2) a ventilated office with one e-cigarette user. Their results showed that exposure to propylene glycol and glycerol may cause bystanders to experience respiratory irritation. The study also suggested that exposure to nicotine could cause heart palpitations and an increase in systolic blood pressure. Due to the presence of TSNAs in some e-liquids, bystanders might have an increased risk of developing tumors, particularly in the car scenario. So, yes, breathing secondhand vape smoke has plenty of health risks.

As it is, lots of teens are taking part in or observing what they call cloud competitions, or gatherings, to see who can perform the coolest vaping tricks. They're promoting them on social media, and some vape shops host them, sometimes offering thousands of dollars in prizes to winners. Imagine the exposure risks in those tightly organized gatherings.

Acknowledging the dangers of secondhand vape smoke, many airlines, restaurants, and other publicly accessible companies have banned vaping, as they did with smoking in the 2000s and 2010s. Many states, cities, and towns have expanded their smoke-free laws to enforce a ban on e-cigarette use in the same places where they forbid smoking cigarettes.

NICOTINE ADDICTION

Nicotine invades every aspect of your life. Addicts physically crave the chemical. Habitual users mentally desire the drug's feel-good effects, such as relaxation and stress relief. The hook can become behavioral, too, triggered, for example, after meals, when with friends, or under stress.

Vaping delivers nicotine incredibly efficiently. Addiction specialists such as Dr. Steven Karp, the chief medical officer at my Breathe Life Healing Centers in West Hollywood, California, worry that vaping is *more* addictive than cigarettes because vape juice often contains higher concentrations of nicotine than cigarettes and your body metabolizes it more quickly.

When you vape, nicotine rushes through your lungs, into your bloodstream, and starts affecting your brain within eight to twenty seconds. It disrupts the normal relationship between a neurochemical called acetylcholine (ACh)—which plays a vital role in muscle contraction, cognition, memory, and more—and its receptors. Think of those receptors as doorbells. Pressing the doorbell outside a home causes someone inside to open the door. But for the doorbell to work, someone must use a finger to press the bell.

Nicotine chemically resembles a finger. Once it binds to the receptor (presses the doorbell), the cell opens the door and lets it in. Imagine hearing your doorbell ring, opening the door, seeing your best friend, and letting him or her inside—only to discover that it's a burglar in disguise.

When nicotine attaches to ACh receptors, it triggers feel-good sensations such as alertness or calmness, focus or relaxation, which makes you want more of it. It also stimulates the release of dopamine in the brain. You associate nicotine use with feeling good, so of course you want more. A similar effect happens when people use cocaine or heroin. In fact, the National Institutes of Health considers nicotine *as addictive* as heroin and cocaine.

Over time, the brain increases its number of ACh receptors, a phenomenon not observed with other addictive drugs. Having more of these receptors intensifies the cravings for more nicotine, which makes trying to quit even harder because those receptors specifically want nicotine. That's the chemical cycle of nicotine addiction.

Conditioning Factors

But people get hooked on e-cigarettes for other reasons, including their environments, social settings, emotions, stress, and other factors. You may puff in certain situations, such as when sipping coffee in the morning, commuting to work, after having lunch with coworkers, or while drinking at a bar. When repeated, these behaviors become wired as cues to your brain to vape and also make it harder to quit. That process is called conditioning.

Conditioning depends on the people, places, and things you associate with e-cigarettes, but the result is usually the same. Put yourself in a vape-triggering situation, and you'll want the missing piece of the puzzle: your e-cig.

Emotional conditioning plays a role, too. Let's say, for example, that you associate chocolate chip cookies with happiness and comfort. The next time you feel depressed, what's a great, easy way to boost your mood? Cookies of course. The more you eat them to make yourself feel better, the more your body will want you to eat them to churn out feel-good chemicals such as dopamine and serotonin. Vaping functions the same way. If when you're down or stressed, puffing lifts you up and makes you feel better, you're going to turn your e-cigarette into a personal coping mechanism.

Defeating these conditioning factors can feel like the hardest part of the quitting process, which is why my program intensively focuses on beating them.

Nicotine Addiction and the Teenage Brain

Nicotine spells trouble at any age, but it's extremely dangerous before the brain develops fully, which doesn't happen until around age twenty-five. That's why scientists agonize about vaping's effects on adolescent brains. Teens are vaping now, but we might not see the worst results until much further down the road.

There's not an easy, ethical way to study precisely what nicotine does to a teenager's brain, but we know that it interrupts its normal function. Research on young lab animals reveals that nicotine can thwart processes critical to impulse control, focus, learning, memory, and even brain development itself. A key problem goes back to nicotine's similarity to acetylcholine in the brain and its skill at fooling those receptors, which actively control the parts of the brain maturing during adolescence.

We don't know for sure, but scientists think that exposure to nicotine as a teen increases the brain-rewarding properties of other drugs, including alcohol, cocaine, meth, and opioids. We do know that we always want more of those feel-good chemicals, so it's easy to understand how amplifying them lays the groundwork for nicotine addiction.

Vape juice contains more than just nicotine, though. Think about bubble gum or cotton candy. Did your mouth just water a little bit? Mine did. Other addiction specialists and I wonder whether these carefully designed flavors offer a dopamine rush of their own. As published in 2018 in *Neuropharmacology*, a team of researchers at Yale investigated this phenomenon. They gave rodents plain and flavored liquids both containing nicotine. The sweet flavoring made the nicotine more palatable and increased the animals' nicotine consumption.

All of which means that quitting nicotine might be harder for teens than for adults. A news story published in *California Healthline* in September 2019 provides evidence for this problem. A young guy began smoking cigarettes in high school, but after hearing that e-cigs were safer, he switched to vaping. Not surprisingly, his nicotine addiction worsened. After a couple of years, he wanted to quit vaping so badly that he turned back to the original problem: smoking. "Juul made my nicotine addiction a lot worse," he told the reporter. "When I didn't have it for more than two hours, I'd get very anxious."

In 2018, *BMJ Case Reports* reported a twist that we saw in Myth 6 (page 15). Teens vaping at a young age are twice as likely to try cigarettes later in life because of nicotine dependency or other social factors. But switching to smoking isn't the answer. The solution is to quit nicotine altogether.

Case in point: encouraged by his parents, Kenny (not his real name), age seventeen, enrolled in my quit program after vaping for three years and puffing whenever he had a free moment. "I was hooked from the end of the first week, and I loved trying different flavors," he told me. "Once I got it going with vape, it was like my puppy dog: always there, in my pocket, in my hands, between my lips, inhaling and exhaling."

Kenny offers a good example of how easily teens can get hooked. Vaping literally rewires their brains. Fortunately he didn't fall prey to other substances. He went through my program and gave up the vape for good.

Withdrawal

With any addiction, withdrawal has both physical and mental components.

Your body reacts to the absence of nicotine in severe ways. A study published in *Nicotine & Tobacco Research* in 2019 examined 109 smokers who had switched to vaping. Researchers at the University of Vermont found that seven days of abstinence from e-cigarettes produced the following withdrawal symptoms: cravings for e-cigarettes, cravings for traditional cigarettes, impulsive behavior, inability to feel pleasure (a common symptom of depression), and mood swings.

Giving up a daily habit triggers a major change in mindset, and it also has an emotional component, as the study above suggests. You might feel defenseless, hopeless, or like you're losing your best friend, and withdrawal can affect your relationships, too. Positive feelings can fuel addiction, but so can a desire to avoid these nasty components of withdrawal. Which is why we'll address them carefully, step-by-step, in the quit program.

You Can Quit

Quitting is a process. It takes desire, work, commitment, and time to move past the cravings and create genuine, healthy alternatives to your chemical dependency.

I'll be honest with you: vaping can be just as hard to quit as cigarettes, if not harder. Maybe you already tried to stop and are struggling. Maybe you feel totally powerless over your nicotine addiction. That's OK as long as you understand that you do have the power to take action. Anyone, no matter how addicted, can quit vaping. Give me twenty-eight days and a willingness to live better, longer, and stronger, and I'll help you do all three by kicking the habit.

Are You Addicted to Nicotine?

Circle either YES or NO in response to the following questions:

Have you ever vaped or used e-cigarettes regularly?
YES   NO

Have you tried to stop but couldn't do it?
YES   NO

If you stopped for a while, did you feel ill or experience withdrawal symptoms?
YES   NO

Have friends or family talked to you or complained about your e-cig use?

YES   NO

Do you hide your vaping paraphernalia from loved ones?

YES   NO

As soon as you wake up, do you feel the urge to puff?

YES   NO

When you leave the house, do you always have your e-cig with you?

YES   NO

Do you find it hard to refrain from vaping in places where it's not allowed?

YES   NO

Scoring

Look over your answers. Assign 1 point to each YES. Add up your score to see where you fall on the following scale:

- 1–2   You don't have a problem yet, but you're playing with fire. Quit while you're ahead.
- 3–5   You probably think that you can stop whenever you want, but it's already too late. You're hooked and you need help.
- 6–8   You have a full-blown addiction, and I can help you break it.

Turn to page 43 and let's begin.

DEAR PARENTS

I f you're the parent or guardian of a teen, chances are that you have already heard the alarm bells blaring about adolescent vaping. You might have attended a school-organized seminar about it. At the Breathe Life Healing Centers, we're hearing that middle-school kids are vaping during and after class. Some high schoolers are vaping whole pods in a single day—roughly an entire pack of cigarettes!—and bragging about sneaking a puff in class without getting caught. We also have treated children who are vaping THC and dabs (marijuana).

Unfortunately our experience isn't unique. It reflects what's happening across the country and increasingly around the world. According to the CDC, more than one in four high school students in America has used e-cigarettes. Here are three stories that put faces on that startling statistic.

For a sixteen-year-old Michigan boy, the scare began on September 17, 2019. Doctors initially diagnosed him with pneumonia, but his condition worsened so quickly that they had to connect him to a special machine called an ECMO (extracorporeal membrane oxygenation) just to keep him alive.

He continued to decline, and on October 3 they transferred him to Henry Ford Hospital in Detroit, where further tests showed enormous amounts of inflammation and scarring in the teen's lungs. Dr. Hassan Nemeh, surgical director of thoracic organ transplants at Henry Ford, had never seen anything like it in his twenty-year career.

The teen was facing certain death from injuries he had sustained from vaping. They put him on the waiting list for a lung transplant on October 8. A week later, he underwent a double lung transplant, the first for someone suffering from EVALI, according to doctors at Henry Ford.

In a statement released by the hospital after the six-hour surgery, the teen's family said:

> Our family could never have imagined being at the center of the largest adolescent public health crisis to face our country in decades. Within a very short period of time, our lives have been forever changed. He has gone from the typical life of a perfectly healthy 16-year-old athlete—attending high school, hanging out with friends, sailing, and playing video games—to waking up intubated and with two new lungs, facing a long and painful recovery process as he struggles to regain his strength and mobility, which has been severely impacted.

Their son celebrated his seventeenth birthday in the hospital.

As of publication, he still is recovering in the hospital, but medical officials plan on transferring him to a rehabilitation facility and expect him to be able to return to school—but he might not make it much beyond that point. For lung-transplant operations, the one-year survival rate is about 85 percent. At five years, only half of recipients are still alive.

"I would expect him to be an advocate to stop this madness," Dr. Nemeh told the media.

One of the most widely reported teen-vaping stories was that of eighteen-year-old Piper Johnson. She first tried e-cigarettes during her sophomore year of high school. By her senior year, she was hooked, going through two to three pods a week.

In summer 2019, the Johnson family piled in a rented SUV packed tight with her belongings for a cross-country trek to get her safely to college. A long road trip has its downsides, but in the Johnsons' case, it may have saved their daughter's life.

"As we began our drive, Piper was coughing and mentioned that it hurt her to take a deep breath," her mother, Ruby, wrote on Facebook. The family made it as far as Greeley, Colorado, where they stopped at a hospital, thinking that Piper was suffering from a simple case of bronchitis. At the hospital, one doctor diagnosed the teen with early pneumonia, while a radiologist initially read her chest X-ray as clear and unremarkable. Confusion abounded, and a proper diagnosis eluded both the medical team and the family.

The situation deteriorated quickly, however, and by the next morning, a CT scan showed what the doctor called diffuse pneumonia, a severe and spreading inflammatory reaction to an allergen in the lungs. That meant that it wasn't occurring in just one area, as is typical for viral or bacterial pneumonia. It was *all over*.

The doctors put Piper on increasing amounts of oxygen along with IV fluids, antibiotics, pain meds, antinausea meds, and a diuretic to help clear the fluid from her lungs. Eventually they transferred her to the ICU. The toxins from vaping had taken a brutal toll on her body, and she was struggling with the lungs of an old, sick woman. The medical team and family had to take extreme precautions to avoid introducing viruses or bacteria that the teen physically couldn't fight. They all wore masks, gloves, and protective clothing around her. Piper cried to a nurse that it hurt badly even to take a simple breath.

Piper Johnson became Colorado's first confirmed case of EVALI, but thankfully she didn't join the ranks of those who have died. She was lucky. After a weeklong stay, the hospital discharged her and expects her to make a full recovery.

Her mother further posted that her daughter is "100 percent owning her choices and has asked me to share her story so that other teenagers can hopefully make other choices."

School friends introduced Anne Peters (not her real name) to vaping in September 2016. She started doing it after class to feel like she belonged, and it completely hooked her. "It was considered cool in my group of friends," she later said.

In January 2017, her parents found vaping paraphernalia hidden in her bedroom, so they knew what she was doing. Even after they confiscated it, they kept finding more under her bed or among the clothes in her closet.

"I realized that she needed professional help to quit," said her mother, Cindy.

Anne's parents sent her to Breathe Life Healing Centers to help her break her vaping habit. She saw red and kicked a hole through her bedroom wall with so much force that she sprained her ankle. She just wanted her parents to stop invading her privacy, stay out of her business, and leave her alone.

At the center, Anne spent twenty-eight days learning and completing the quit program in this book. "I was there for Juuling. There were some people there for coke, some for weed, some for pills. I realized I was a nicotine addict. The hardest part about quitting was the withdrawal," she told me. "You feel trapped, scrambled, and very scared."

But Anne made it. She quit, and since then she has become an antivaping advocate. She first spoke about her experience at her own high school, and the reaction from her classmates bordered on ridicule. But recently, as news of vaping-related illnesses and deaths has become commonplace, she finds herself answering questions from previously skeptical friends and others who tell her: "I really need to stop, but I don't know how. How do I stop?"

Anne formed a support group to help them. Now she travels to schools all around California with her mother, and they share her story and explain how kids in each audience can find the help they need to quit.

These three stories underscore that we're facing a critical teen health crisis. Vape devices, flavors, and marketing specifically target teens and young adults, so the e-cig industry will continue to grow unless we do something about it at both ends of the equation. What can you do with your child? Here are some important, lifesaving suggestions.

Set the Example

We learn language, beliefs, habits, mannerisms, and countless other behaviors by watching others, particularly parents, siblings, peers, and partners. That process is called modeling.

In a now-classic study, psychologist Albert Bandura had kids watch adults punch and kick those inflatable figures with weighted bottoms that bounce back when you strike them. Later, when left alone with the dolls, the children turned into pint-sized prizefighters. They pummeled the dolls, just as the adults had done. The adults modeled the behavior, and the kids repeated it. If you want your teen to behave in a certain way, make sure that he or she does as you say and as you do.

Set a positive example by remaining substance free. Addiction has a genetic component, so children from families with a history of substance abuse may have a greater risk of developing a nicotine habit. If you smoke, be prepared to answer the question: "You smoke, so why do you care if I vape?"

You might respond with something like: "I wish I had never started. I don't want you to make the same mistakes that I did." But that isn't going to cut it. You saw right through that line when you were a kid, and so will your kid. If you do smoke, vape, or abuse another substance, make a plan to quit together and help each other achieve your goals.

Know the Signs

Vaping can be hard to detect because, unlike smoking, the aerosol dissipates quickly and leaves little scent or residue on breath, hair, or clothes. But the presence of several or more of the following clues may suggest that your kid is vaping.

Unusual Nosebleeds: Vaping dries out the mouth and also dehydrates the delicate membranes inside the nose. When these become too dry, they can crack and bleed. If your child doesn't have a history of nosebleeds but suddenly they start happening frequently, that might offer a sign that he or she has started vaping.

Avoiding Caffeine: As they develop, teenagers need a lot of sleep, and their sleep patterns differ significantly from younger kids and adults. As a result, teens often start drinking coffee to realign their systems with the rest of the world. But remember, nicotine is also a stimulant. Vaping nicotine plus drinking caffeine can trigger anxiety attacks and severe mood swings. Because of that, vapers tend to reduce their caffeine intake. Take note if your latte-loving kiddo inexplicably starts skipping the coffeemaker or café.

Abnormal Thirst: Vaping is a hydroscopic activity, which means that it dehydrates the skin of the mouth and throat. The propylene glycol in vape juice also pulls water molecules from the mouth and nose. Both of these chemical reactions leave vapers with dry mouth. Consequently, their bodies crave lots of liquids to combat dehydration. If your child starts chugging water or other fluids for an extended period of time (and is peeing more frequently), he or she may be vaping.

Craving Flavor: Moisture in the mouth helps improve the taste of food. When the mouth and tongue dry out, they can't taste as well. With routine vaping, food tends to taste bland, a condition called vaper's tongue. If your teen had a sensitive palate or a sweet tooth but all of a sudden starts salting meals heavily or eating a lot of super-spicy foods, that could be another indication.

Unfamiliar Items: E-cigarettes come in many shapes and sizes. Lots of them look like USB drives, and many have batteries that require charging or other parts that you may not recognize, including wires and small containers called pods or cartridges that contain vape juice. If your teen brings home a new, odd-looking, high-tech device, ask about it. If you find strange items in his or her trash can, ask casually what they are.

Addiction Behaviors: Here's where it starts to get tricky. The signs of a nicotine habit can look a lot like the normal behavior of your average teenager, particularly irritability, frequent snacking, and changes in sleep habits. As a parent, you have a baseline sense of what's normal for your kid. Significant deviations in those behaviors and a meaningful increase in random coughing could be a warning sign.

Unusual Acne: The surge of hormones that triggers adolescent development also causes many teens to develop oily skin. The bacteria that cause acne thrive in that oily environment, and everyday stress can cause breakouts, so developing acne itself isn't a clue. But vaping can cause a dramatic increase in facial acne because vape juice contains noxious chemicals harmful to the skin.

Secretive Behavior: Teens are naturally secretive creatures. Withdrawing into personal space helps them establish their independence and self-sufficiency. But there's a difference between wanting some alone time and acting like a spy. If your kid won't emerge from behind closed doors on reasonable occasions, opens windows at odd times, or makes unusually frequent trips outside or to the bathroom, he or she may be trying to conceal a vaping habit. Also watch for attempts to hide small electrical devices, unfamiliar charging cords, and the colorful plastic caps that come with pods or cartridges.

PAVe the Way

Parents Against Vaping e-cigarettes (PAVe) started with three women: Dina Alessi, Meredith Berkman, and Dorian Fuhrman. Among them, these moms had nine kids, ages seven to nineteen. They joined forces in spring 2018 after they discovered that their teen sons were Juuling. The women researched the behavior and quickly realized that the use of flavored e-cigs—Juul in particular—had reached epidemic proportions. They founded PAVe as a grassroots response to vaping and its dangers, and the organization educates parents and empowers them to take action.

Their message: "We will not allow Big Tobacco 2.0 to take advantage of our kids, turning them into an entire generation of nicotine addicts!" PAVe provides educational materials and other resources that you can access at Parents AgainstVaping.org.

Talk. Teach. Test.

Even if your teenager hates or challenges everything you say, you still remain a powerful influence in his or her life. Opportunities to discuss vaping with your teen can present themselves in many ways: posts on social media, stories on TV, passing a vape shop, or seeing someone vaping. Whatever the situation, have a conversation rather than a confrontation. Listen rather than lecture! Here are some of the most effective ways to steer kids away from vaping:

Establish a Vape- and Smoke-Free Home: Prohibit family and friends from smoking or vaping in your home or other personal space.

Start Early: Talk about vaping and smoking when your kid is in kindergarten—and don't stop. Teach the truths of vaping. Keep the conversation going as he or she gets older. When in doubt if your kid is vaping—test for the presence of nicotine!

Keep Conversations Safe: Avoid direct questions that sound accusatory, such as *"Are* you vaping?" Instead, use a more casual, nonjudgmental approach, such as: "I've been hearing a lot about vaping lately. How popular is it at school? Has anyone you know gotten sick from it? What do you think about it? What do you imagine it does to a person's lungs?"

Have Answers: One of the simultaneous joys and horrors of being a parent is that you never know what's going to come out of your kid's mouth. If he or she asks about vaping, respond honestly but don't go over the top trying to frighten them. Most kids love nothing more than challenging their parents' boundaries. If you answer calmly and matter-of-factly, he or she is more likely to pay attention and listen to what you say.

If your teen parrots one of the myths mentioned earlier, share the truth and the facts to support it.

He or she might say: "Everyone's doing it, who cares?" and the honest answer is that *you* care because no one else in the world cares as much about your child as you do. Make sure that he or she understands that.

Rebel with a Cause

It's hard to watch kids make bad decisions, but sometimes they need to do that to learn valuable lessons. It's important for you to voice your concerns along the way, but bad-mouthing your teen's friends might push him or her closer to them. At the same time, it's equally important that your child knows that he or she has to earn your trust.

If you know that your kid's friends are vaping, be specific and direct: "I don't like that X and Y are vaping, but I know that you won't because I trust you." Always give your kid a positive reason to do what you say—in this case, earning your trust and reaping its rewards—rather than a negative, such as the thrill of breaking the rules and getting away with it.

If that doesn't work—and it won't for every kid—a tougher course of action is separating your child from the bad crowd, which you should do based on direct observation rather than suspicion. Kids need clear boundaries, so if you forbid yours from hanging out with a particular bad influence or group, make sure that the consequences are clear from the beginning, then follow through on them.

The flip side of this coin is to weaponize your teen's rebellious nature against him or her. Teenagers naturally organize themselves into like-minded cliques, but they hate feeling like sheep. If your kids say something like, "Everyone's vaping, who cares?" point out that, if everyone's doing it, then they're just blindly following the herd and not making their own decisions about their own bodies.

Some Great Reward

In middle school, the dad of one of my best friends offered her a thousand dollars if she didn't try a cigarette before age twenty-one. She didn't, and, on her twenty-first birthday, her dad paid up. The deal worked.

According to a 2019 study from Britain, published in the *Cochrane Database of Systematic Reviews*, monetary incentives for quitting smoking do help smokers kick their habit and remain smoke free. For the study, investigators analyzed thirty-three randomized and controlled trials. The studies included more than 21,600 people in eight countries and looked at whether financial incentives, such as cash payments, vouchers, or the return of money deposited by participants helped them quit smoking. The researchers found that after six months or more, people who received financial rewards were about 50 percent more likely to have quit smoking than those in the control groups.

We don't yet know whether the same type of reward system will work for teen vapers, but it's certainly worth a try. Create timed incentives to keep your teen focused on not vaping. What matters most to your kid? Art, money, music, nature, sports, travel, video games—whatever it is, make sure that he or she has a positive reason to avoid vaping. After all, it's pretty hard for anyone to argue with: "My parents are paying me not to vape!"

Slide into Their DMs

To help teenagers quit vaping, Truth Initiative created a first-of-its-kind program that offers support via texting. Kids who text "quit" to (202) 804-9884 will receive daily text messages offering assistance and guiding them to resources designed specifically for them, including encouragement, tips, and tools for how to quit. If your child won't do it, consider texting it for him or her.

Don't Scare Them

As a motive for personal change, fear is about as successful as nagging. Neither works very well, and fear in particular *rarely* works with kids. When faced with all the negative results, they run further into denial and dig in their heels. Your teen already knows that you disapprove of vaping, so stern lectures and scare tactics won't help. You're not going to hear, "Gee, thanks for pointing that out again!"

Kids need to hear words of love and encouragement. Let them know how important they are to you, and make sure that you show it, too. Tell them that you want them in your life for the rest of your life. Describe activities that you want to do together in the future. The promise of quality time together is stronger than the fear of getting sick, so that's what you need to emphasize to sell the quit. Then, instead of punishing them, calmly connect them with the science. Explain that nicotine is highly addictive and especially dangerous when the brain is still under construction, until age twenty-five.

If your child goes through this program, tolerate the frustration, moodiness, and snarkiness and continue to give your full support through the rough patches of quitting an addiction as well as the achievements.

Intervene

In an adult, stubbornness and tenacity can lead to success and triumph, but some kids are more willful than seems humanly possible. If your child continues to vape despite a calm, loving approach, positive reinforcement, and clear, reasonable boundaries with fair consequences, it can feel absolutely maddening.

Most people, including kids, don't change on their own. They need external encouragement and sometimes lots of it. The Appendix details how to undertake a loving intervention, but here's a preview with some additional details that apply especially to teens.

You know that you can't do it on your own, so you need the help of trusted people who matter to your kid, such as siblings, cousins, friends, teammates, coaches, teachers, aunts or uncles, and others. Make sure to include a mix of nonvapers and ex-vapers, people your child's age and other adults whom your child admires or respects. Getting support from others is vital.

Gather this Quit Team with your teen and offer him or her an invitation to change in which everyone participates. The three steps of the conversation should follow the same basic pattern as your one-on-one conversations:

1. Again, kids need to hear love and encouragement. The Quit Team should explain first how important your teen is to each of them and what positive activities they want to do with him or her in the future.
2. They each should give a recent example or two of the negative impacts that your child's vaping has had on each relationship and how vaping will prevent the previously stated positive activities from happening.
3. The Quit Team should commit to helping your kid kick the habit and offer whatever support he or she needs, with accountability to include nicotine test strips (readily available online) to test your kid's urine or saliva.

Be there for your teen and help him or her however you can, including as a guide through the quit program in this book. Again, be supportive and patient. Love him or her unconditionally and always make it clear that you're frustrated with the vaping behavior and not your child.

Part Two

The Program

STEP ONE
PLAN YOUR QUIT

Days 1–7

You know that vaping isn't good for you, but you still haven't managed to stop. That's what we do with much of what we know: little to nothing. It's like the story of the turtle who fell into the pothole.

A turtle was ambling down a country road when she fell into a muddy pothole. She strained her stubby legs, but she couldn't free herself. Soon her friend rabbit hopped by and offered to help.

"It's no use," said the turtle. "Nothing will work. I'm stuck."

Other friends passed her way and also offered to assist, but the turtle refused their help. She believed that the muddy mire was her destiny, so she retreated into the familiar protection of her shell. As she lamented her situation in darkness, she heard a loud noise. Peeking out, the turtle saw a tractor rumbling toward her down the road. Suddenly the little reptile flipped herself out of the pothole to the safety of the side of the road.

Like the turtle, we choose not to change—to flip ourselves out of life's potholes—until we hurt badly enough or face truly imminent danger. But this fable demonstrates that when you have the proper motivation, you can accomplish the seemingly impossible.

Quitting anything requires dedication and a plan. The following steps and activities will give you the strength and resolve to quit vaping even when you feel helpless and hopeless. They will move you forward because they direct your psychological momentum toward quitting, give you the time that you need to prepare, and help you commit yourself to the task. The power to change your life for the better begins in these early stages. So in the spirit of getting ready to flip yourself from the pothole of vaping, imagine the next week as the time you're putting your quit in motion.

In this step, you will:

- Set your quit date.
- Envision becoming an ex-vaper.
- Taper off nicotine.
- Complete a nutritional detox.
- Assemble your support team.
- Defeat your doubts.
- Learn and practice the H2M technique.

Day 1

Set Your Quit Day

Today you choose your quit date. You're ready to do what it takes to achieve the goal of kicking your vaping habit. This date becomes a calendar promise between you and your family, partner, friends, God, the universe, or any and all of the above. It's the date that you decide your vaping days are over.

Select the date, seven days from now—Day 7 of the plan—on which you'll stop vaping. You choose the day, and you make it official. Each of the days between now and then will prepare you for that day, giving you guidelines and helping you gradually reduce the number of times you vape each day. By working toward your Quit Day, you're giving yourself the freedom you need to prepare yourself to quit vaping.

For years, medical officials advised smokers and other nicotine addicts to quit cold turkey, meaning instantaneously and using just willpower, rather than tapering. Research shows that if you can quit on your planned Quit Day, you have a greater chance of quitting for good. A study, published in the *Annals of Internal Medicine* in 2016, followed seven hundred British smokers who wanted to kick the habit. Researchers divided them into two groups: one group received a quit day, while the other group was instructed to taper gradually. The study found that one month after their Quit Day, 49 percent of participants in that group weren't smoking anymore, compared with 39 percent in the taper group. Six months later, a gap between the groups still held: 22 percent of the Quit Day group weren't smoking, compared with 15.5 percent of the taper group.

Setting a Quit Day worked for Caroline, age thirty-four. After smoking two packs of cigarettes a day for fifteen years, she switched to vaping. She liked that she didn't smell like a chimney anymore, nor was she suffering from as much anxiety. Still, Caroline worried that she had traded one bad habit for another. Which of course she had. Caroline decided to quit vaping. I explained that she needed to select a quit date in the near future, at which point she would vape no more. Here, in her own words, is what happened on that day:

"Usually, one of the first things I do when I wake up is reach for my pod. I just loved to vape with my morning cup of coffee. On my Quit Day, I was determined not to do it. So I got out of bed, made my coffee, and sat down to watch the news—all without my vape. At that point, I'd usually be enjoying a few satisfying draws.

"I continued following this routine along with the program. To my surprise, I felt pretty good without the vape. This went on for a couple of weeks, I was happy, and soon I felt as if I had never vaped. The process of stopping with a quit date was very effective. When I finally stopped vaping, I was surprised to discover that I felt not just relief but happiness."

Selecting a Quit Day works.

Accountability is also key. Let your loved ones know what you're doing. We are creatures of habit and connection. When you share this important decision and powerful plan, your chances of success skyrocket because we change best together. Your Quit Day is a cause for celebration. On that date, you and your loved ones will celebrate your commitment to live a better, longer, stronger life.

Day 1 Assignment

- ❏ Select your Quit Day for seven days from now: ____/____/____
- ❏ Memorize the date, put it in your calendar app, circle it on every physical calendar that you own, and write it down on your Quit Calendar (page 156).
- ❏ Start your Quit Kit (page 159), which will guide you through important exercises to reinforce your resolve to stop vaping.
- ❏ Write out your Quit Date Promise (page 160) and don't forget to sign and date it.
- ❏ Take a picture of your Quit Date Promise and share it with loved ones and on social media.

Teen Talk: U

As we've seen, it might be tougher for teens to quit than adults because nicotine radically rewires young minds. Teenagers are more vulnerable to addiction because their brains are still developing, which makes them more likely to fall into substance abuse. They also probably don't see the dangers of vaping because they like to fit in and they love to rebel.

Help your teen set his or her quit date with a texting service. Thousands of kids who vape are signing up for these programs, especially after hearing that vaping is making so many other teenagers ill, including their own friends.

A 2019 article in Apple News posed the logical question: "But do the students think it will make a difference?" One high school freshman replied: "I do, yeah. For a lot of people actually. I've known kids who have stopped vaping because of it."

Truth Initiative offers one of the best texting services available. It's free, organized by age group, and gives teens and young adults helpful recommendations. They can enroll anonymously by texting "quit" to (202) 804-9884. If your teen resists the idea, consider texting it for him or her.

Social media is what users make of it, so of course some people spread pro-vape propaganda on it. But, like these texting services, it can play a key role in helping teens to quit vaping. Monitor the accounts that your child is following and make sure that he or she is viewing and interacting with antivape content or at least not following anyone promoting the activity.

Day 2

Envision Becoming an Ex-Vaper

Visualization, or guided mental imagery, has profound benefits when practiced regularly. The process is simple: you form positive images in your mind in order to work toward a goal.

When you picture something you want, you're conditioning your neural networks—the nerve cells that link your body to your brain—to recognize what you want to achieve. Athletes use this technique all the time to boost their confidence, strength, and performance. While focusing on all of their senses, they visualize and mentally rehearse their entire performance in vivid detail. Carli Lloyd, a star player on the U.S. women's soccer team, uses visualization and credits it with helping her on the field. While training for a World Cup game against Japan, she visualized herself scoring four goals. In the game, she kicked three balls into the net—the first woman in World Cup history to do so.

Your brain is powerful and trainable. Visualization will enable you to tap into the power of your subconscious mind and help you see yourself becoming an ex-vaper. It also intersects with the Law of Attraction, which states that you have the power to attract into your life whatever you think about. Positive thoughts attract positive results; negative thoughts invite negative outcomes. It may sound like nonsense, but it's not. What we believe, we can achieve.

Today you'll start visualizing yourself as an ex-vaper. The following exercise will help you create that pathway in your neural network.

Visualization Exercise

1. Sit in a quiet place, in a comfortable position, with your eyes closed.
2. Keep your spine straight and breathe deeply as you relax your body.
3. Focus on your goal: to quit vaping.
4. Imagine your future. You have achieved your goal of vaping no more. How does that look? Watch yourself moving through your day in as much detail as possible, engaging as many of the five senses as possible. Picture the answers to each of these questions:

   - What are you wearing?
   - What are you doing?
   - What sounds do your inhaling and exhaling make?
   - What are your surroundings?
   - What do you hear?
   - What can you smell?
   - If you're eating or drinking something, how does it taste?
   - Who are you with?
   - How do you feel?

5. If doubts come into your mind, acknowledge them. Now turn them into blue balloons and watch them float away or crumple them up like a sheet of paper and throw them in the garbage. As you watch them disappear, repeat one of the mantras on page 74.

This technique gives you a powerful tool for overcoming your nicotine addiction. Begin by visualizing for five minutes a day, then gradually increase to ten minutes. Use this technique every day during your quit and then whenever you need or want it.

Experiment with visualizations, too. Envision the same activities over and over, which can help cement success in your mind. Try different scenarios for variety if that keeps you more engaged—or do both and see what technique works best for you.

Another tool that harnesses the power of visualization is a Vision Board. It can be as small as a sheet of paper or as large as a poster, but it will help you see the changes you want in your life.

Day 2 Assignment

❏ Do your first Visualization Exercise for five minutes.
❏ In your Quit Kit (page 159), write down how your life will look as an ex-vaper. If you have trouble with the Visualization Exercise today or on any other day, read aloud to yourself what you write.
❏ Take the Commitment Quiz (page 162).
❏ Create your Vision Board (page 163) and place it somewhere meaningful where you will see it every day to remind you of what you are trying to achieve.

Teen Talk: The Focus Challenge

Addiction gravely impacts the ability to focus, especially in teens. Kids in the Breathe Life Healing Centers program tell us that, at first, vaping makes them more alert and attentive, but then their attention spans decrease. One high schooler had no trouble sitting through midterm exams, but after vaping for six months, he couldn't sit still because of the cravings, couldn't think of the answers to test questions, and just fidgeted.

Visualization requires focus, so it may work better for adults than teens. If your child is having trouble doing the Visualization Exercise, taking the Commitment Quiz, or creating the Vision Board solo, get involved. Ask the questions first, have your teen answer you aloud, and then prompt him or her with those same answers for writing down in the Quit Kit. Lend a hand with gathering and printing source material for the Vision Board, but make sure that your child is making the decisions about what to put on it.

If you're having trouble facilitating an open conversation about vaping, try taking your teen to see his or her pediatrician. We know that with cigarettes, if your physician tells you not to smoke, that doubles your chances of quitting. Teenagers love to challenge their parents, but they tend to show more respect for and listen better to other authority figures. The pediatrician or pulmonologist talking about vaping, without Mom or Dad in the room, might work.

Day 3

Replace and Taper

Nicotine replacement therapy (NRT) works by delivering measured doses of the substance into the body through a gum, inhalator (inhaler), lozenge, patch, or spray. Nicotine continues to enter your system, but you're not taxing your lungs with the other toxic ingredients in vape juice. NRT doesn't help with social or emotional triggers—which we'll tackle later in the program—but it can help reduce your cravings and withdrawal symptoms so you can focus on conquering your underlying addiction.

Medical professionals have been using NRT successfully for more than thirty years, and lots of solid science shows that NRT increases your chances of recovering from nicotine dependence. A 2018 review of 136 studies that involved nearly sixty-five thousand people, published in the *Cochrane Database of Systematic Reviews*, shows that NRT increases the rate of quitting by more than 50 percent!

Note: Teens (see page 57) without parental support or women who are pregnant or nursing should *not* use NRT.

To start reducing your physical dependence on nicotine, I recommend over-the-counter nicotine lozenges or nose spray. Both deliver nicotine and give your lungs a much-needed break. NRT does not replicate the inhale-exhale behavior of drawing on an e-cig, which of course you want to stop doing. Possible side effects include coughing, irritation of the mouth or throat, and a runny nose. Rarer problems can include headaches, anxiety, and a racing heartbeat, which have to do with the nicotine rather than the spray or lozenge.

All NRT products are available over the counter without a prescription to those over twenty-one. I cannot guarantee that NRT will work for you, but NRT has helped hundreds of thousands of people quit or significantly reduce the amount of harm that vaping is doing to their bodies.

If you decide to use NRT in your quit, you need to talk to your health-care provider to determine the right doses and the proper timing for tapering to avoid severe withdrawal symptoms. On our Quit Vaping Facebook group we offer help videos. Always follow the instructions *exactly*. Make sure that you understand the tapering process, dosages, and timing. If you experience any significant side effects, see your health-care provider right away.

When you combine NRT with the other steps in the program, it can help you quit.

Day 3 Assignment

❏ Look into NRT today. Which product do you think might work best for you?
❏ Review the Quit Vaping Facebook group's How To video library.
❏ If you think NRT will help you, schedule an appointment with your health-care provider to establish dosages and a timetable. When you have those, put them in your calendar app, on any physical calendars that you have, and on your Quit Calendar (page 156).

Teen Talk: NRT Red Flag

From studies on smoking, we know that NRT generally works better for adults than for adolescents. Adults can buy most NRT medications over the counter, but a minor needs a prescription. Because NRT contains nicotine, teens should *not* use it unless under the close supervision of a parent and pediatrician. According to the Mayo Clinic, "Additional clinical trials are warranted to evaluate whether NRT provides benefit to adolescent smokers." Remember, nicotine can damage still-maturing brains, so proceed with caution.

Day 4

Nutritional Detox

You've been inhaling nicotine and other toxins multiple times a day, every day. It's not healthy, but your body knows the routine. Quitting upsets that routine, which can come as a shock to your system. You can combat that shock by giving your body the proper nutrition that it craves.

People addicted to nicotine have lower levels of:

- Antioxidants, such as beta carotene, vitamin E, and selenium, which help defeat damage-causing free radicals.
- Vitamin C, which supports the immune system and prevents organ damage.
- Vitamin D, which promotes bone health and the immune system. (Nicotine addicts have a greater risk of developing osteoporosis and of breaking bones.)

Adjusting your diet and taking the right supplements will improve your energy levels, concentration, mood, and overall well-being. When you feel better, you do better, and that includes achieving your quit.

Here are my detox guidelines:

Avoid Mucus-Producing Foods: Some mucus in the lungs is normal, but chronic mucus can block the airways and cause breathing problems. People who vape already risk developing excess mucus, so it's important not to add to it. One way to do that is through diet. Certain foods and food groups may promote excess mucus: chocolate, dairy (cheese, milk, ice cream, yogurt), fast food, and processed meats. Steer clear.

Go Alkaline: As you might remember from chemistry class, acidity and alkalinity fall along the pH scale. The lower the pH, the more acidic; the higher the pH, the more alkaline. Pure, distilled water sits right in the middle of the scale at 7.0.

Alkaline foods, such as fruits and vegetables, help detox the body, whereas acidic foods can trigger an inflammatory response. Acids also can turn into free radicals, causing tissue damage. Eating alkaline foods can soothe inflamed tissue, heal ulcerations, and enhance cellular function.

These foods make your body more acidic, and you want to stay away from them:

- Alcohol
- Artificial sweeteners
- Caffeine
- Dairy
- Fatty meats
- Processed foods, such as packaged snacks, hot dogs, cold cuts, and frozen dinners
- Refined grains and nutrient-poor carbs, such as sugary boxed cereals, white bread, white pasta, and white rice
- Sugar and sugary foods, including sodas

You don't have to avoid all these foods all the time, but you definitely should reduce your intake of them. Remember, think: more good, less bad.

To go alkaline, eat at least five servings of fruits and vegetables a day, especially leafy greens and low-sugar fruits such as avocados, berries, and citrus. (Citrus fruits contain acid but, once digested, have an alkaline effect on the body.) These foods contain lots of disease-fighting antioxidants, which can curtail the production of mucus and phlegm in the body and keep them from congregating in your lungs.

Plant proteins, such as beans, nuts, seeds, and tofu, are great for the body and are gaining in availability, popularity, and variety. (They're also much better for the environment than animal protein.) If you prefer animal protein, choose a variety of lean cuts of meat and enjoy them in moderation. For example: chicken or turkey three times a week, eggs a few times a week, fish a couple of times a week, and red meat just once a week. Eggs and fish in particular contain lots of choline, a B vitamin that boosts brain power and may help with withdrawal symptoms.

Remember, too, that sugar is its own kind of drug. We often use it to elevate our dopamine levels, even though we don't know we're doing it for that reason. Sugar is also very acidic to the body.

If you can make your meals about 80 percent alkaline, you're doing great. You'll feel the benefits in improved energy levels, better sleep, and increased vitality.

You can measure your alkalinity levels with urine test strips available online or at most drugstores. Use them on your second pee of the day (to bypass acidity accumulated overnight) and aim for a more alkaline reading. What you eat can change your pH for the better.

Cruciferous Vegetables: These veggies are good for you and associated with a lower risk of lung cancer. Eat them raw or cooked.

- Arugula
- Bok choy
- Broccoli
- Brussels sprouts
- Cabbage
- Cauliflower
- Collard greens
- Horseradish
- Kale
- Radish
- Wasabi
- Watercress

After you quit vaping, eating more of these veggies can help reverse the damage. Pretty amazing, right?

Spice It Up: Gingerroot has well-documented antioxidant, anti-inflammatory, and anticancer properties. It also helps break down mucus and remove it from the body. Grate it raw on salads, cook with it, or make a delicious ginger tea with lemon and a little honey.

Other herbs, such as eucalyptus, orange peel, oregano, and peppermint, also promote lung health. Make them into teas, cook with them, or take them as herbal supplements.

Hydrate: It's important to drink plenty of water every day. Water flushes residual nicotine and other waste from your body, and staying well hydrated will make you feel better overall, which will make it easier to tackle any withdrawal symptoms that you might experience. Drinking water may help reduce cravings as well. Drink at least eight 8-ounce glasses each day and consider buying filtered alkaline water, which should have a pH of 8.0 or more. Alkaline water contains many mineral antioxidants, and research has shown that drinking it increases overall health and well-being.

Supplement Your Diet: These supplements are useful for detoxing from nicotine and lessening withdrawal symptoms. Consider taking:

- A multivitamin, which contains lots of antioxidants that help reduce the toxicity of nicotine and alleviate irritation from free radicals.
- Vitamin B, which nicotine depletes in the body. The different types of B vitamins include: thiamine (B_1), niacin (B_3), choline (B_4), pyridoxine (B_6), and cobalamin (B_{12}). Vitamin B_3 helps dilate constricted blood vessels, and B_{12} can help reverse cellular damage. A good B-vitamin complex will supply all of these B vitamins in one pill.
- Vitamin C, which, in addition to supporting your immune system, can help reduce nicotine cravings.
- Omega-3 fatty acids, typically made from fish oil, which promote whole-body health. Researchers in Brazil gave nicotine-dependent study participants three grams of fish oil three times a day for ninety days, and they gave a control group mineral oil as a placebo. After treatment, the fish-oil group showed a significant reduction in their levels of dependence. If you're vegetarian or vegan, flaxseed, chia seeds, and walnuts contain lots of omega-3 fatty acids.
- Tyrosine, an amino acid that reverses lung damage, supports heart health and serves as a building block for dopamine.

Vaping Vitamins?

Several companies sell vape juice that contains vitamins, herbal supplements, and essential oils. One company advertises that its B_{12} vaporizer contains "10 times the amount found in a typical B-12 shot" and shows it next to fresh fruits and berries—none of which contains vitamin B_{12}.

Very little research has studied whether vaping your vitamins is either safe or effective, but we know that heating vape juice can produce new chemicals not in the original liquid. I prefer to get my nutrients from food first, then supplements, and *never* from vaping. Our lungs are designed to breathe clean air, and that's it. Love the lungs you're with.

Day 4 Assignment

❏ Clear your pantry and fridge of sugary, processed zero foods (because they have zero nutritional value) and any other overly acidic or mucus-causing foods that you should be avoiding.

❏ Stock up on lots of alkaline foods and start eating them.

❏ Buy alkaline water and start drinking it.

❏ Purchase the recommended supplements and start taking them.

Teen Talk: Feed Them Well

Adolescents love fast food, soda, and other processed food, and they don't always eat at home, where you can monitor their intake. Some suggestions to help them eat well:

- Model good nutritional habits. Don't skip meals or overindulge on fast food or other junk food. Teens follow good examples rather than rules.

- Don't make a big announcement about eating healthier; just introduce healthy foods gradually. You still control a lot of meals, so add a fruit or vegetable—or an extra—to every meal.

- Add extra veggies to casseroles, pizza, sandwiches, smoothies, soups, stews, and other dishes.

- Gradually get rid of junk food around the house and replace it with a bowl of fruit or raw nuts for snacking.

- Eat together as a family. Doing that three to five times a week has many proven benefits, including better nutrition, increased academic performance, improved relationships, and lower rates of risky behavior (such as vaping). Family meals don't always have to be dinner, either. Saturday breakfasts or weekend lunches work great, too.

Day 5

Assemble Your Quit Team

We humans are communal creatures by nature. We thrive when we work together and share our experiences and abilities. We need people in our lives who care about us, with whom we can share our problems, and who will support us when we need it. The buddy system works. That's why you shouldn't keep your problems to yourself. If you need help, ask for it. With strong, positive support around you, your commitment will be much easier to sustain and your quit will go more smoothly. So you need to assemble a Quit Team.

Start with your family, particularly your spouse or partner, parents, or siblings. A huge body of literature supports the involvement of family members in recovery. On your team, you want someone who supports your quit without judgment, demands, or abuse of other substances.

Also look to your peers, specifically your closest nonvaping friends or friends who have quit successfully. They can offer inspiration and hold you accountable. In some research studies, participants who had a Quit Buddy were three times more likely to quit successfully. If someone you know wants to give up vaping, too, suggest quitting together.

At the same time, you need to break ties with your friends who vape or at least avoid them when they're puffing. Steering clear of vape-using friends will help you change your identity from vaper to ex-vaper. It may be hard to withdraw from a social circle that encourages or tolerates the habit, but you need to resist the temptation. If necessary, develop a plan to avoid that group.

You already shared the good news that you're quitting. Remind your friends and loved ones that you're serious and then plan activities with them that will help you not vape. Give them the power to stop you from asking for a puff in moments of craving. It might annoy you when they say no or try to interrupt you, but you'll thank them in the long run.

Consider joining a support group. They come in various forms: some highly structured, others more informal. They usually meet on a regular basis—once a week, once a month—in the homes of members or in a more public location, such as a community center. Whatever the arrangement, they all have the common goal of joining together people with similar experiences, who, by sharing, can gain strength and hope from one another. Think of it as just a bigger version of the buddy system.

Online groups have advantages, too. The biggest is their round-the-clock availability. Support, encouragement, and inspiration are only a click away, day or night. Look around to see whether any online communities appeal to you. On Facebook, my friend, colleague, and ex-vaper Mackenzie Phillips and I have a vibrant support spot. Join us there in the group Quit Vaping with Brad and Mack.

You also might try connecting with a treatment professional or therapist. They offer compassionate, nonjudgmental support that goes beneath the addiction and addresses the issues that might have led to it. Their understanding and insight often serve as a critical motivator for successful recovery.

Whichever path works best for you, lean on those who love you, people who have defeated a similar problem, or professionals. Ask for support, accept it, and count your blessings, because life *is* getting better.

Day 5 Assignment

❏ In your Quit Kit (page 159), name at least five people to your Quit Team who want you to stop vaping. Can one of them act as your Quit Buddy?

❏ Write out a list of statements or questions (page 166) that you want to hear from your Quit Team and then share that list with them so they know how to help.

❏ If you need to avoid a vape-friendly social circle, develop your Escape Plan (page 166).

❏ Create your Activity List (page 167) to do with friends and family to help you avoid temptation and then firmly schedule those activities.

❏ Do your Visualization Exercise (page 52).

Teen Talk: Parental Support

Sometimes the best support is your time. Special activities are great, but spending quality time together can be as simple as exercising, going to church, going for a walk, working on a hobby, or even just *being* together. Whatever the activity, do something with your teen that makes life fun or more fulfilling.

Quality time also means being emotionally available. Your teen may not want to hang out with you, but that doesn't mean that he or she isn't paying attention. Show your love and concern with a pat on the back, a hug, or a smile. Offer a sympathetic, listening ear and make sure that your child knows that you love him or her and that you aren't sitting in judgment. Stay off your device and practice being devoted company.

Day 6

Defeat Your Doubts

Self-doubt—that troubling, persuasive voice in the back of your head—can block you from seizing important opportunities and make recovery harder than it should be. By giving you excuses that follow the path of least resistance, it allows you to remain hooked to your habit and to opt out of quitting. So how can you overcome a lack of conviction and belief in yourself in order to move forward?

First, know that you're not alone. Everyone has self-doubts—*everyone*. Here are the five most common self-doubts that I've heard over the years and the truths that will show you how to handle them. These truths represent rational wisdom, the realities that your crippling self-doubts are clouding reality. Read through them and see which ones sound most familiar. You may relate to one, some, or all of them.

Doubt: The cravings will be too much for me to handle. I won't be able to quit.

Truth: Quitting causes cravings, but you can conquer them.

Withdrawal isn't easy, and sometimes the cravings will feel intense. The process will cause temporary mood swings, but as long as you recognize that they're temporary, you can remain in control and continue to make good decisions. This is where the help of your Quit Team matters. If you feel the dragon of addiction taking flight, alert your team, pause, and breathe. You can do this. Remember, thousands of people have felt exactly the same and still quit successfully.

Doubt: Just the thought of trying to stop makes me nervous. I can't handle the anxiety.

Truth: Quitting can feel emotionally overwhelming, but achieving your goal will bring you newfound calm.

Everyday life can be super stressful without the added worry of quitting nicotine. Avoid anxiety-provoking situations as much as you can and alert trusted coworkers so they can support you during your quit. If it gets really bad, tell someone on your Quit Team what's making you feel anxious and why. Don't keep your doubts inside, or they'll seem worse than they really are. Let them out into the light. Just saying them aloud might help to brighten the worst darkness of your thoughts. If you have a diagnosed anxiety disorder, talk to your doctor or therapist about techniques that you can use to help you through the worst of it. Avoid benzodiazepines, which are useful at helping deal with anxiety but also are high risk for those with addiction history. "Benzos" are highly addictive and dangerous.

Doubt: If I try to quit, I'm going to fail, which will make me feel depressed.

Truth: Depression is part of the roller coaster, but quitting will make you feel happy.

Depression is the flip side of anxiety. Nicotine chemically lights up your brain like a Christmas tree. Pulling the plug on it is going to make you feel darker, but, again, that feeling is only temporary. For many vapers, the habit itself feels like a best friend, the one who's been there through thick and thin, ups and downs. It's a reliable source of comfort, so of course the thought of quitting is going to affect you. It's hard to lose a friend! Remember who your real friends are: your Quit Team cheering you on to stop vaping for good.

If cutting back on nicotine makes you feel seriously down in the dumps, definitely investigate nicotine replacement therapy. People who use NRT are twice as likely to quit successfully *and* they're less prone to depression. If you have diagnosed depression, talk to your doctor or therapist about what you can do to get through this darkness.

Doubt: Trying to stop vaping fries my concentration. Quitting will short-circuit my brain.

Truth: Nicotine affects your brain, so quitting will cause an inability to focus, but it's temporary.

Quitting might make you feel distracted and slow. Withdrawal can feel like you're drowning in mud. It seems as though the feeling will never end, but soon your ability to concentrate will return *and* improve. As with anxiety, NRT will help you conquer this side effect of quitting. While you're at it, try meditation (page 110) or yoga (page 113). Both are mindful practices that will help you improve your ability to focus. Also, the more exercise (page 90) you do during your detox, the more quickly the nicotine will leave your system. Other helpers to post-acute withdrawal syndrome include a hot bath, massage, and even acupuncture. Once your body expels the chemical, quitting becomes an issue of mind over matter. Plan to do the work, and then work the plan.

Doubt: I don't want to quit because I like the flavor, and I'll miss it.

Truth: Vape juice might taste good, but quitting will taste better.

Vaping dulls taste buds, so the intense chemical ingredients of vape juice might taste good, but everything else probably tastes a little gray ("vaper's tongue"). Think about how great your favorite foods and drinks will taste again when your taste buds return to normal.

Addiction clouds thinking on truth here. No matter how unsure you feel about kicking your habit, remain steadfast, remember that countless others have done it before you, and don't let your doubts get you down. Believe in yourself because you have everything to gain by kicking your vape habit.

Day 6 Assignment

❑ In your Quit Kit (page 159), identify which doubts resonated most strongly with you and then defeat them.
❑ Which of those doubts is the strongest? Write a break-up letter to your biggest doubt.
❑ Do your Visualization Exercise (page 52).

Teen Talk: How to Reason with Your Child

Try to see vaping from a teenager's perspective. Most of them know that opioids and hard street drugs are horrible, but they don't see vaping as that dangerous. If you explode with anger, they're going to think you're overreacting, making a big deal over nothing, and they're going to rebel, which is what teens do best. One of their doubts is that vaping isn't nearly as bad as everyone says it is. Your job as a parent or guardian is to convince them that the truth is, well, true.

But you can't use scare tactics. Have a calm, honest conversation with your child. Share what researchers have discovered and encourage your teen to quit on his or her own terms. Don't blindly berate or punish. Find out what doubts he or she has about vaping or quitting and pursue them. If those doubts are accurate, reinforce them appropriately. If the doubts are false, gently guide your teen to the truth.

Day 7

Practice H2M and Begin NRT

It's Quit Day! Today you become an ex-vaper. Congratulations!

Now you're ready to learn a powerful technique that will help you reduce your vaping habit. It's called Hand to Mouth (H2M), and you'll use it to replace the physical act of vaping. H2M is another form of replacement therapy.

In addiction, every time you vape, you grab the device, activate it, put it to your lips, and inhale a potent dose of nicotine. That series of actions has become a habit in and of itself. To stop vaping successfully, you need to delete this programmed habit from your behavioral circuitry. You regularly upgrade programs on your computer or apps on your smartphone. Now it's time to upgrade the operating system in your brain.

Vaping creates an oral fixation and a physical contract with your hand and mouth. H2M gives you a healthy alternative that mimics some of the routine of vaping, reduces anxiety, and helps you commit to your quit. Just ten cumulative minutes of H2M will help you beat the average nicotine craving. How great is that? Here's how it works.

H2M

1. Make a fist with your dominant hand, the one you use to hold your vaping device.
2. Bring your fist to your mouth, with your closed thumb and forefinger against your lips.

3. Inhale deeply through your nose.
4. Exhale through your clenched fist.
5. Repeat five times.

This practice creates a comforting oral experience that replicates the physical behavior of vaping without relying on nicotine or other dangerous chemicals. As you repeat this technique, focus on your breathing. Feel it fill your lungs and warm your fist.

When you feel comfortable with the steps above, add a mental mantra or affirmation when you exhale. This mantra can be any word or phrase that you like and will help carve a new groove in your brain that overwrites the vaping pathway. Repeat it in your mind each time you exhale. When quitting smoking, I chose "Long Live Me" as my mantra because to me quitting represented more life, more love, and a healthier body.

Here are some additional words, phrases, and affirmations that you might try.

Mental Mantras

Breathing in change brings me joy.

Energy and freedom.

Freedom.

I feel better with each breath.

I've dumped my vape kit for good.

I hold peace in breathing as intended.

I shall vape no more.

I'm an ex-vaper.

I'm happy and relaxed.

I'm healthier by choosing clean air for my lungs.

I'm in control.

I am sturdy.

I'm vape free.

Life, love, health.

My lungs are clear and strong.

You can repeat the same mantra over and over again, try different mantras for variety, or pick a couple of favorites to use when fighting cravings.

When you practice H2M, you're inhaling change and a new life and exhaling your nicotine addiction and the past. Doesn't that feel good?

If people ask what you're doing, don't be shy. Tell them what you've learned: that you have a new tool to help you quit vaping.

One of my clients, Marty, thought he was doing himself a favor by switching from more than three decades of smoking to vaping. After a few months, he still couldn't make it to the mailbox without stopping to catch his breath.

When he learned H2M, he had that "aha!" moment: "I hadn't realized that, with smoking, then with vaping, I had a thirty-five-year hand-to-mouth habit that made quitting extremely difficult. This step got me over it fast. Almost two years ago, I was so addicted that I thought I'd never be able to quit. Today I am totally vape- and smoke-free." H2M coupled with beginning NRT (the gum, patch, lozenge, or nasal spray) are key to starting your stop. You are ready.

Day 7 Assignment

❏ Practice H2M at least three times today and use your
   NRT no matter what.
❏ In your Quit Kit (page 159), generate more mental man-
   tras that can help you focus on breathing through your
   cravings.
❏ Do your Visualization Exercise (page 52).
❏ Make sure your vape equipment is out of reach and in
   a dump.

Teen Talk: Modeling

As we saw in "Dear Parents," kids tend to learn most effectively
by mimicking adult behavior rather than by listening to a lecture
or reading a book. If your child feels stupid or foolish doing H2M
on his or her own, show how it's done to model the behavior
and make it feel less awkward. Also work with your teen to find
the right mental mantra that will make H2M that much more
effective.

STEP TWO
MANAGE YOUR CRAVINGS
Days 8–14

Cravings are the biggest obstacle to kicking addiction. One minute, you're doing fine, feeling healthy, happy, and proud. Then, out of nowhere, you feel like you can't go another second without a puff. People always say, "One day at a time," but sometimes it's more like one second at a time. When cravings rise like a powerful wave, you need to ride them out instead of letting them overwhelm you. Step Two is all about learning how to do that.

First, congratulate yourself on making it this far. Seriously. Stand up—yes, *right now*—and cheer for yourself out loud. You've earned it! You're putting in the time and effort to change and heal. You've got this!

In this step, you will:

- Continue to use H2M and NRT.
- Double-check that all vape devices are at the dump.
- Conquer your emotional triggers.
- Vary your routine to avoid vaping.
- Sweat out the nicotine.
- Monitor your internal dialogue.
- Recognize your progress.
- Pursue your passions.

Day 8

Clean House

Addressing a deep emotional house cleaning is ahead, though let's double-check you have made your home, your car, and your bag reflective of an ex-vaper. You can't vape if the opportunity doesn't exist. Reducing your exposure to vaping products helps you defend yourself from temptation and makes it harder to lapse. Today you're going to double-check that all physical traces and reminders of vaping from your environment and anywhere that you vaped are a thing of the past.

The psychological term for these reminders is cues, which trigger or prompt your desire to puff. Cues can be internal or external, and they're extremely powerful. Internal cues are generally emotional; for example: anger, anxiety, boredom, depression, fear, sadness, or stress. That desire to vape stems not from your body's physical dependency on nicotine but from your mind. We'll talk about managing those internal cues later in the program.

External cues come from your environment. These tangible triggers also stimulate your urge to vape. Examples of external cues include:

- Places, such as your car, home, office, or school, where you have a history of vaping
- Vape ads on TV or online
- Seeing vaping products
- Spotting a vape shop

- Watching people vape
- Someone offering you a puff

If you've tried to quit before, you know how strong these cues can feel. You'll face temptation when friends or family vape around you, seeing other people doing it, and in places where you used to do it. You might also miss the actions themselves, such as holding the device in your hand, putting it between your lips, and pulling a drag from it. When that happens, keep practicing H2M (page 73).

But you also need to eliminate the external cues that are triggering you. This step, cleaning house, has nothing to do with willpower. White-knuckle determination will get you only so far, and you have a very limited amount of it. Using willpower alone to resist cravings is like trying to hold a beach ball underwater. Sure, you can do it for a little while, but it takes an enormous amount of strength, and eventually up pops the ball.

If you do lapse, you might experience feelings of shame, self-condemnation, or guilt: *Why can't I have more self-control? I'm never going to be able to do this. I might as well just give up now.* None of those thoughts is productive, and nothing is wrong with you. You are *not* a failure. You don't need willpower to master your cravings. You need to reengineer your environment for success.

They might not seem external, but also remember to eliminate online cues, as seventeen-year-old Dan (not his real name) did. "I was constantly on my computer or iPhone, Googling stuff about how safe vaping is. I wanted affirmation, but deep down I was kidding myself," he told me. "Part of my quit on this day was to resist the urge to Google pro-vaping info. I also unsubscribed from all my vaping sites. It was a great move for me."

In an environment without drugs, any addict can conquer his or her addiction. So if you want to quit vaping, you need to rid your environment of all reminders of the activity. It's much easier to vape in public than to smoke, so controlling external cues can prove more challenging for vapers. Nonetheless, limiting them will decrease your opportunities to vape and set you on the right track.

Day 8 Assignment

❏ Continue with H2M (page 73) and your NRT (page 55).
❏ Use your Clean House Checklists (page 170) to purge all traces of vaping from your life.
❏ If you have a car, have it detailed, take it to a car wash, or give it a thorough clean yourself.
❏ Wash any clothes or linens that you often wear or use while vaping.
❏ Do a deep clean on the places you like to vape in your home.
❏ Do your Visualization Exercise (page 52).

Teen Talk: Hiding Places

Most teens don't even like to clean their rooms, and they certainly don't want to divulge their hiding places for contraband paraphernalia, so you've got a challenge. If they won't even pick their up their dirty jeans, how are you going to make sure they clean house?

First, asking them to ditch the vaping stuff from their bedrooms isn't too much to ask. They live in your house, so they have to follow the house rules. If you don't allow vaping in your home, then they can't keep any of the supplies or accessories. That's a fair and reasonable expectation.

But they also don't have to reveal their hiding places to you. Ask them to remove all of their vaping items from their rooms, using the checklist on pages 170, and put all of it in a bin or box that you provide. Let them know, too, that you will be making periodic walk-throughs to make sure they are following your rules.

Teens have a lot of hiding spots and stashes that may not be in their rooms. An obvious spot is their lockers at school. Here's where it helps to communicate with school officials to encourage locker checks. It might surprise you how many schools are tackling the teen vaping crisis. Some schools have installed technology that detects where and when kids are vaping at school. When the detectors sense a certain chemical, an alert goes straight to school officials. Make sure that your teen knows that's a possibility. Talk. Teach. Test. That's what you do to leverage change and verify abstinence.

Day 9

Emotional Cues

Your feelings themselves can point you to vape if you regularly puff in response to anger, fear, guilt, joy, loneliness, or other emotions. You can use vaping to enhance a good mood—feeling excited, happy, or satisfied—or escape a bad one—feeling anxious, bored, or depressed. Correctly identifying your feelings is critical to your quit because you need to reprogram yourself away from vaping as a coping mechanism or crutch.

Putting a name to how you feel is the first step toward mastering your emotions and using them for good. In my work with thousands of clients over the years, I've identified and organized the most common emotional cues into this baseline feelings table.

Emotion	Result When Embraced	Result When Redirected
anger	rage, stress	motivation, power, action
fear	worry, panic, paranoia	wisdom, self-protection, good instincts
guilt	immobility, numbness	justice, good values
joy	hysteria, mania	passion, hope, love
loneliness	isolation, helplessness	independence, self-reliance
pain, hurt	misery, hopelessness, depression	healing, discovery, growth
shame	worthlessness, self-pity	humility, humanity

As you can see, all emotions can lead to negative or positive feelings. You have the power to decide which. By first acknowledging your emotions, you can then respond to them rationally and redirect them in the positive ways listed in the third column above.

We are creatures of habit, and more often than not we react to similar situations in similar ways. When mad, for example, some yell. If you're feeling sad, you might isolate yourself from friends and family. The next time you're feeling particularly emotional, try responding differently. If you're feeling lonely, make a point to see, call, or text your Quit Buddy or someone on your Quit Team.

It also helps to develop specific mantras for specific emotions. Take a look at the Mental Mantras (page 74) again and see which ones might work for the emotions that you're feeling.

If you need something more active, try one or more of these positive, healthy actions that you can do to help yourself feel calmer and more secure.

Self-Care Activities

- Make yourself a cup of decaf coffee, tea, or cocoa.
- Take a shower or bath.
- Meditate.
- Stretch.
- Listen to some soothing music.
- Read a book or listen to an audiobook.
- Call or text your Quit Buddy or a member of your Quit Team.
- Watch a favorite movie or TV show.

- Go for a walk.
- Do a favorite hobby, such as painting, playing an instrument, or cooking.

Your emotions are valid, so you should acknowledge them, but don't let them control your life. As you redirect them, you are reprogramming them to have less power over you. When you create new emotional responses, the old ones will fade, and you will succeed in your quit.

Day 9 Assignment

❏ Continue with H2M (page 73) and your NRT (page 55).
❏ In your Quit Kit (page 159), identify which emotions or feelings are triggering you to vape and why.
❏ Create emotional mantras that will help you redirect and reprogram those cues. Repeat the mantras when negative feelings overwhelm you.
❏ Select the Self-Care Activities that will help you feel calmer and more secure.
❏ Do your Visualization Exercise (page 52).
❏ Practice H2M (page 73).

Teen Talk: Managing Emotional Triggers

Like anyone, it's common for teens to want to vape to escape bad moods or to prolong good ones. But teens often have trouble figuring out what they're feeling because their emotional awareness is developing along with their bodies. As a parent, here's how you can help your teen manage his or her feelings without reaching for the vape.

Allow Breaks: Taking a breather from an upsetting or stressful situation can help your teen calm down. Take a walk around the block, listen to some favorite music, or find a quiet spot to breathe.

Move Around: Physical activity is a great way to handle and release overwhelming emotions. Invite your kid to the gym with you, shoot some hoops, or go for a walk, jog, or bike ride together.

Promote Healthy Habits: Make sure your teen eats a balanced diet, drinks lots of water, and gets enough sleep, which help both body and mind feel good.

Give Rewards: Remind your teen about the rewards coming for reaching milestones and quitting successfully. Focusing on something that he or she wants can act as a mood-busting distraction.

Make Resources Available: Enlist someone on your child's Quit Team to help him or her talk it out. If you think that he or she might need more professional help, consider a therapist.

Day 10

Change Your Routine

In addition to environmental and emotional cues, part of the challenge of quitting has to do with our routines. A routine, sometimes called a behavior chain, is any series of actions or habits that we do frequently, automatically, and in a particular order.

A typical behavior chain for someone who vapes might be: come home from work, grab a snack from the fridge, turn on the TV, sit down, and vape. Each activity forms a link in the behavior chain and points to the end result of vaping.

One of my clients, Vic, turned one of his vaping routines into a hobby. After coming home from work every day, he mixed different flavors of vape juice like a mad scientist. "It was nuts, but that was my routine," he told me. "Get off work, experiment with mixing juices, vape them like crazy. The problem with this routine is that it got all-consuming. I wasn't spending time with my wife or kids. Honestly, this obsession was wrecking my family life. Ultimately I had to create new, healthier after-work activities like helping my wife around the house, doing stuff with my children— basically substituting family things for a really unhealthy and stupid hobby."

To change your negative routines, you have to shake things up with chain-breaking activities. Do you usually eat lunch at your desk and then head outside to vape? Have lunch in the cafeteria with coworkers and then walk with them back to your desk. Do you like to vape before cooking dinner? Chat with a friend or spend time with your kids instead. Not only will you avoid vaping, but you'll focus on why you wanted to quit in the first place.

Here are other simple ways that you can break behavior chains and thus change your vaping routines:

Vaping Routine	New Routine
on waking	Take a shower right away.
with coffee or tea	Change what you drink or where you drink it. Sit in a different room or with different people.
at your desk	Reorganize your desk or its location. Fidget with something, such as a stress ball or finger spinner.
after meals	Drink water, brush your teeth, or go for a walk or bike ride.
after work	Exercise or meditate. Pursue creative projects or a hobby. Go to a bookstore or see a movie. Listen to music; read a newspaper, magazine, or book; or play a video game.
before dinner	Eat earlier or later. If you often cook at home, eat out or order in. If you frequently eat out, cook at home.
with alcohol	Try a different drink and hold it in your vape hand.
while thinking	Practice H2M, breathe deeply, or stretch.
as a reward	Have a healthy snack, such as a handful of nuts or a piece of fruit.
with vapers	Chew gum or drink water. Avoid vapers altogether if you can.
while reading or watching TV	Rearrange your furniture, organize paperwork, fidget with a stress ball, or do some stretches.
before bed	Sip a warm drink. Read a book. Chat with someone on your Quit Team.

This table addresses your vaping routines specifically, but other habits might be tempting you. Change your normal travel routes so that you don't pass any vape shops. Where do you usually go to vape? Go somewhere else instead. If possible, use different exits and entrances and avoid places where others regularly vape. Spend as much of your free time as possible in places where vaping isn't allowed. Change the channel if you see vaping commercials on TV or close your browser if you spot them online.

You also can break the behavior chain by undertaking an incompatible activity; for example: biking or swimming. It's extremely difficult to vape while holding on to handlebars, and it's impossible to do it underwater. To be effective, chain-breaking activities must be readily available, and they have to compete with the urge to vape. Changing your routine avoids the trigger. Breaking the chain overwhelms it.

Eliminating self-destructive routines and replacing them with good habits will help you defeat your cravings and increase your chances of quitting successfully.

Day 10 Assignment

❏ In your Quit Kit (page 159), identify other routines that culminate in vaping and replace them with new habits.
❏ Do your Visualization Exercise (page 52).
❏ Practice H2M (page 73).

Teen Talk: Shake It Up

Kids need routines to help them navigate the world, so changing them can feel disruptive and prove harder to accomplish than for adults. It's also more difficult to get teens to adopt good new habits. As usual, incentives and rewards help. If you're still struggling, have your kid focus on how his or her vaping routines have made life worse. In a calm, nonjudgmental tone, ask:

- How much time do you spend vaping every day? What else would you rather do with that time?
- How much money do you spend on vaping? What else would you rather buy with it?
- What can't you do anymore that you used to enjoy?

Help them see for themselves that their vaping routines are changing their lives in negative ways and that they have other options.

Day 11

Exercise Your Quit

Stress is one of the most common triggers for vaping. One of the best ways to combat stress is to exercise. Physical activity of any kind—even if it's moderate and you don't sweat or pant—can improve your brain chemistry, making you feel happier and more productive. Exercise releases endorphins, feel-good hormones that boost your mood and kill your cravings. Exercising also distracts you from the temptation to vape.

A 2017 study published in *Experimental and Clinical Psycopharmacology* reviewed the benefits of physical activity in treating nicotine addiction. Exercise:

- Reduced cravings for nicotine.
- Reduced cue-induced cravings.
- Lengthened time between cravings.
- Helped people withdraw from nicotine.
- Helped people stay abstinent from nicotine.

When you think about exercising, what comes to mind? Long-distance running? Doing jumping jacks in a class? Lifting at the gym? Those are all great examples, but they aren't your only options, nor may they work for you. You might enjoy biking, dancing, gardening, paddleboarding, surfing, swimming, or even just taking a long walk. Take a boxing, Pilates, spin, Tai Chi, yoga, or Zumba class. Not for you? Try basketball, golfing, soccer, tennis, or another sport.

What kind of exercise should you do? Whatever you enjoy—but you need to have fun doing it! If it's not enjoyable, it's not sustainable.

Mark, an eighteen-year-old vaper, didn't exercise much until his best friend gave him a free pass to a kickboxing class. He went to the studio, and, to his surprise, he really enjoyed it. "I punched out a lot of stress, and it felt good," he said.

Since that initial visit, he has donned the gloves and helmet four times a week. He feels stronger—which keeps him motivated—and loves the camaraderie of the class. Kickboxing also gave him a keen awareness of how vaping compromises his breathing and strength. "If I vape the day of a workout, I can really feel it in the studio. I wear out too fast, and I can't push myself like I want to."

His enjoyment of kickboxing ultimately helped him kick the habit. Today Mark is vape free and in great shape to boot.

You don't have to choose a structured class like Mark did. You just have to find something you like that gets you moving. Some people don't like to exercise or can't find the time, but if you have time to vape, you have time to do something active. If you get bored easily at the gym, try watching one of your favorite shows or listening to a motivational playlist or podcast.

Note: vaping tends to inflame lung tissue, so exercise caution—literally. Hard cardio, such as running, spinning, or swimming, might be too much for your lungs until you've been vape free for at least a month. Start with gentler exercises for now, and always consult your health-care provider prior to starting any exercise program.

Get moving at least three times a week, for twenty to thirty minutes each time. Stay consistent and try to increase your amount of physical activity with each session. Also plan to exercise when your cravings hit hardest. Studies show that nicotine cravings skyrocket in the morning, dip at midday, and peak again in the evening.

If you need some extra motivation:

- Schedule regular workout times and set reminders for them.
- Establish a fitness goal, such as being able to do five pull-ups in a row, running a 5K, or losing five pounds.
- Reach out to your Quit Team for support and consider exercising with a buddy.
- Hire a personal trainer who will help keep you motivated and accountable.

Remember, think fun!

Day 11 Assignment

- ❏ In your Quit Kit (page 159), list the exercises, sports, or other forms of physical activity that appeal to you.
- ❏ Schedule your exercise activities and stick to them by putting them into your calendar app or writing them in your calendar. Do this *every* week.
- ❏ Do your Visualization Exercise (page 52).
- ❏ Practice H2M (page 73).

Teen Talk: Athletic Performance

Teens generally have higher energy levels than adults, which you can harness to help them quit. But remember that vaping makes it harder to breathe. If your teen is an athlete or physically active, look for opportunities to discuss how vaping might be affecting physical performance. Have energy levels dipped? Is it harder to breathe? Be ready to listen rather than lecture.

The teenagers who use Truth Initiative's free texting service also worry about how vaping affects their health and athletic abilities. The organization provided NBC News with an anonymous sampling of reasons that young people are giving for wanting to quit. Examples include:

If I get caught, I'm off the team.
I don't want my lungs to hurt. I want to be healthy.
I can't stand the anxiousness.
It makes me feel depressed and unmotivated.

Day 12

Monitor Your Messaging

We all have a running commentary in our heads. It's that internal voice that helps us process new information, make decisions, and formulate plans. Take a moment to think about how your inner voice sounds. Is it kind, loving, and supportive, or does it like to beat you up and drag you down?

The way you speak to yourself, your self-messaging, determines how successful you'll be at achieving your goals. What are you telling yourself about yourself? What does your inner voice think of you? Stalactites and stalagmites form in caves over many years as tiny drops of water deposit minerals and sediment on top of one another. That's how your self-messaging forms who you are and how you see yourself. If you're constantly telling yourself that you're a failure, your inner dialogue is ensuring that you won't kick your fix.

Your self-messaging both carves and follows some pretty deep grooves in your brain. You probably barely notice it on a conscious level. Time to start paying attention. Here's how:

- Take the time to listen carefully to what you're saying to yourself. Meditation is a great way to tune out distractions and focus on your inner dialogue.
- If your self-messaging sounds like a bitter critic, give it a name and an identity that you can dismiss easily: "Oh, that's just X piping up again because Y."
- What advice would you give to a friend in the same situation? Give that advice to yourself.

- Concentrate on past accomplishments and successes. What achievements make you feel most proud?
- Build yourself up with messages, such as: *I believe in myself. I am smart, strong, and talented. I can do this.*

Repetition is all it takes to create a good new habit. Repeating new behaviors creates new beliefs, which lead to new feelings, which trigger new actions. One of the best ways to anchor your new beliefs is to say them aloud. Speaking them and hearing them trains that voice in your head—in two ways simultaneously—to speak more kindly and supportively to you.

It also helps to do it in the mirror. It might feel hokey, but you don't have to believe what you're saying when you do it. You just have to say the words aloud to yourself. Relax into it, and let the process do the work. Try some of these:

"I can beat this craving."

"Breathing well makes me feel good."

"Honesty is the key to my progress."

"I have a loving team that wants me to succeed."

In order to reach a goal, you first need to believe that you can achieve it. You have the power to choose the tone and content of your self-messaging and make sure that it feeds you a steady stream of encouragement and positive energy whenever you need it.

Day 12 Assignment

❑ In your Quit Kit (page 159), write down the five most common thoughts you have about yourself and rewrite the negative ones into positives.

❑ Do your Visualization Exercise (page 52).

❑ Practice H2M (page 73).

Teen Talk: Self-Talk

Adolescents can be their own biggest critics. They hear all kinds of negative commentary every day, but sometimes the worst thoughts come from inside their own heads. Here's what you can do to help your kid think positively and be a better judge of his or her self-worth.

Let Them Brag: Instead of bringing up that D on that test or that they overslept (again), ask questions that lead them to praise their accomplishments: "Did you help anyone today?" "What did you do really well today?" "What made you feel proud today?" "What was the best compliment you received today?"

These questions prompt their developing brains to focus on positives, and they hear that you're encouraging them, which they also need. Bragging like this is beneficial because it slowly builds a good sense of self-worth and self-esteem. Remember to focus on accomplishments rather than innate characteristics, which are harder to control or change.

Emphasize the Small Stuff: Tell them when you're proud of them. Put that last report card on the fridge. Praise how well they're doing in sports, in school, or how helpful they are around the house.

Encourage Realistic Goals: Setting and reaching big goals, like graduating from high school and getting into college, helps teen brains develop properly, but those goals can feel overwhelming sometimes. Help them set smaller, intermediate goals, such as going one day without vaping, completing that 5-page paper, or being able to jog a mile without stopping. When they reach those goals, help them celebrate.

Day 13

Recognize Your Progress

You're nearly two weeks into your quit, so thirteen is your new lucky number. Pat yourself on your back for all the progress you've made. Be extra kind to yourself today, too.

Maybe your quit is feeling tough. If so, read Days 9 through 11 again, and review your Quit Kit from the beginning. Remind yourself how to get through the tough spots, how to stay strong, healthy, and engaged. Pause today to think about three things: your health, your money, and your time.

After you quit, your body purges nicotine from your system in one to three days and other nicotine-related chemicals after ten. So you already made it past the hardest part. Good job! Think about all the healthy new tissue that your body is regenerating. How do you feel physically? When you're not fighting a craving, are your moods better? Do you feel stronger? Do you have more energy? Can you breathe better? Stick with your NRT and keep practicing H2M.

Now let's think about the money. Calculate how much you haven't spent on vaping in the last two weeks. Multiply that number by 26. That's how much you'll save in a year, and it's a decent chunk of change, right? What are you going to do with all that cash? Save it, invest it, or treat yourself or a loved one? Start thinking about a special reward for yourself on the first anniversary of your Quit Day.

Time is the most precious asset of all because once it's gone, you can't get it back. Think about how much time you've saved by not sitting or standing around puffing on a vape pen. By quitting, you've just added years back to your life. What do you want to do with all that time?

Day 13 Assignment

❏ In your Quit Kit (page 159), reflect on all of the good progress that you've made so far.
❏ Do your Visualization Exercise (page 52).
❏ Practice H2M (page 73).

Parent Talk: Go Easy on Yourself

This one's for you. If your kid vapes, you haven't failed as a parent. You aren't a bad parent or a bad person. Hang in there. It's hard, but kids can kick the habit, and you can help. You're already reading this book, which is a great first step that proves that you care.

Take vaping as seriously as any other addiction and sympathize with how hard it must feel to quit. Some kids have rough physical and psychological withdrawal symptoms, and they might lapse. That's OK. Don't panic. It happens, and it's not the end of the world. Your job is to help them get back on their feet and keep trying. You helped them learn how to walk, how to talk, how to tie their shoes, how to read, how to ride a bike or swim. This might feel harder because the stakes are higher, but it's the same thing. You can help them do this, too.

Day 14

Pursue Your Passions

Any kind of addiction erodes your discipline, enthusiasm, and focus. Some addiction specialists think that this decrease in focus on what really matters in life can keep people enslaved to substance abuse. Take the case of Portugal.

More than twenty years ago, that country had one of the worst drug problems in Europe. One in ten people there had fallen into heroin use: bankers, cabbies, carpenters, farmers, salespeople, socialites, students, tailors—everyone. People were using on the street, in public squares, by the side of the road. Crime rates shot through the roof. Not a day passed without a heroin-related robbery or mugging.

Government officials formed a national panel to figure out how to solve the crisis. First, the panel recommended decriminalizing everything, from cannabis to crack, which helped destigmatize substance abuse so that users felt less ashamed for needing help and more comfortable seeking it. The panel also recommended taking all the money the country was spending on arresting and imprisoning drug users and using it instead to reconnect them meaningfully with society.

Dr. João Goulão led that second effort. He wanted every addict in Portugal to wake up with something to do every day. He wanted people to have productive activities to do instead of getting high. The government subsidized housing and jobs for addicts. If a mechanic developed a drug problem, government officials approached a local garage, asked it to employ him for a year, and the government paid half of his wages. The results proved extraordinary: The country's drug use dropped by an astounding 50 percent, and every study showed that addiction rates were decreasing.

My friend Mackenzie Phillips, star of screen and stage, is a daughter of John Phillips of the hit singing group the Mamas and the Papas. As can happen with the children of popular entertainers, she got into drugs and alcohol at a young age and struggled for a long time. She also smoked for forty years. "I loved smoking, or at least loved the hit the nicotine gave me every time I raised my hand to my mouth to inhale," she told me. "My mom had smoked, and she was such a lady. I loved being like her when I started at thirteen years old. I would steal them [cigarettes] from both my folks. They were easy to come by, and readily available.

"I did quit over the years, from time to time, but always found it agonizing, the cravings and emotional highs and lows I would suffer when not smoking. Smoking gave me a great fix."

In recovery for many years, Mack recognized that she had an addiction to smoking. To quit, she switched to vaping. "I kept telling myself it was better than smoking, yet I knew it was awful for me. It was a brutal, awful, humiliating experience, I must say, the powerlessness I felt in being unable to unburden myself from it."

Mack completed my program, is vape free, and, in the process, found a new passion to pursue in her life. She works as a counselor at the Breathe Life Healing Centers.

Nicotine addiction reprograms your brain to focus on nicotine at the expense of everything else, and the act of vaping also takes you away physically from other healthy, enjoyable activities.

Using the lessons of Portugal and Mackenzie Phillips, think about how you can live more passionately. Spend time today considering what, other than vaping, you love to do. What excites you? What lights that fire in your blood? What do you most look forward to doing? Passions change over time, so don't worry if you're not sure. Think about what you loved doing in the past. Maybe it's experiencing art, listening to or playing music, spending time in nature, playing or watching sports, traveling, playing video games, or something else entirely.

Day 14 Assignment

❏ In your Quit Kit (page 159), list the activities or involvements that you used to love doing or still do and make more time for them in your life.
❏ Do your Visualization Exercise (page 52).
❏ Practice H2M (page 73).

Teen Talk: A Passionate Life

One of your jobs as a parent is helping your kids discover and embrace a passionate life. Teenagers love to throw themselves into activities they enjoy and to learn more about how different parts of the world work. It helps them form a positive identity and become adults. One of your goals is to help them find good, healthy passions to pursue. Here's how you can help make that happen.

Let Them Be Themselves: You may want your teen to become a doctor, lawyer, or professional athlete, which would be great, but what does your kid really want to do—right now and in the future? We as parents always want great things for our children, but your hopes and dreams for your child might not fit with who he or she is or, worse, feel like a straitjacket. Give your teen the space to figure this one out alone.

Meaningful Work: Have an ongoing conversation about how following a passion can create a meaningful, rewarding, stable life. Talk about careers and jobs as more than just a means to make money. If they do what they love and work smart and hard, the money will follow.

Plenty of Time: In high school, students often hear questions about what they want to study in college or what career they want to pursue, but a lot of them don't even know what they want for dinner or what to do this weekend. Reassure them that they have time to figure out what they're passionate about. There's time to explore new subjects and develop new interests, and it's OK if those interests change over time.

Talents and Abilities: Teenagers are still learning about themselves, so they might not have any clear passions yet. If that's the case, one way to tackle this issue is to ask: What are you good at, and, in that space, what do you like doing? Is your kid great at fixing things? Good with animals? Maybe she has a gift for leadership, or maybe he's a great dancer.

Encourage your teen to try lots of different activities, no strings attached. Check out local camps, clubs, community centers, online courses, part-time jobs, and teams to see what sparks an interest. Something will stick. The more exposure your kids have to the world, the better they'll understand themselves.

Then, when something good does stick, encourage it—even if it's not your cup of tea or your kid isn't great at it. Adolescence is when kids start becoming their own selves, and you can't stand in the way. Also, with practice, they can develop an aptitude or strength for whatever is striking a chord.

What if your kid wants to quit? Remember, no strings. Make sure that he or she gave it a fair shot and then move on. It's OK to drop something if it truly doesn't resonate.

STEP THREE
LIVE YOUR QUIT

Days 15–21

You've exhaled your past, and now it's time to live your new life. The road ahead still has some bumps and pitfalls, but you've come too far to quit your quit. Take courage and get ready for the freedom that awaits. You're ready for this.

Beneath all the discoveries, hurdles, lessons, and triumphs, your body has been changing. Cravings might nudge you, but now you can push them away much more easily than during week one. Your lungs are breathing better, your heart is pumping healthier, and your body is becoming stronger. The odds that your quit will succeed increase every day. Today you enter week three and embrace your future.

In this step, you will:

- Learn how to avoid social triggers.
- Use meditation to curb cravings.
- Stretch yourself and try yoga.
- Beat your negative beliefs.
- Prepare a relapse prevention plan.
- Check up on your health.
- Reward yourself.

Day 15

Social Triggers

When people vape at a bar, concert, or work, they're following what addiction specialists call a social trigger. These occasions usually include other people who also vape, and the situation itself prompts a desire to puff. If you vape and find yourself around other vapers, you're more likely to feel the urge, especially if those other vapers belong to your social group.

You have control over your own actions, but you can't control what other people do. You may find yourself unable to avoid a family member who vapes, for example. To eliminate these social triggers and reduce situational urges, take the following actions.

At Work

Avoid the smoking or vaping area. Stick to places where you won't face temptation. When you see your vaping buddies head outside, change what you're doing. Get up from your desk and fill your water bottle, do some quick exercises or stretches, or grab a healthy snack or pop a piece of gum in your mouth. *Don't* follow them outside and go for a walk around the block. Keep them out of sight to keep them out of mind. Cravings can feel more powerful when your blood sugar levels are running low, so snacks such as fruit, nuts, or low-sugar yogurt are helpful.

Bring a discreet hobby or fidget device, such as a stress

ball or finger spinner, to work. You need to take breaks to stay focused, but you also need to replace vaping as your go-to break activity. When you feel the urge, focus on something quick that you enjoy doing. Play a short game of solitaire or sudoku, knit a few rows of yarn, read a couple of pages of a book, or sketch something interesting in the office. Keep your vape hand occupied.

At Parties and Events

If people are going outside to vape, stay indoors and keep your line of sight focused in the opposite direction. Volunteer to help the host by serving appetizers, making sure guests have drinks, or helping in the kitchen. Again, keep your vaping hand occupied. These activities will keep you busy and help keep your mind off vaping. Hang out with nonvapers to reinforce your resolve. If you can, bring a guest—ideally someone from your Quit Team—who doesn't puff. If people are vaping at the event itself, excuse yourself and take a walk around the block.

At Bars

Alcohol affects your ability to make good decisions and it reduces your inhibitions. For many people, alcohol itself becomes a trigger, so avoid bars with a dedicated smoking area—or altogether—until you're confident you won't vape while there. If you do want or need to go to a bar, go *only* with nonvaping friends and deputize one or more of them to keep you from relapse.

Traveling

You may want to cut loose or try new behaviors or activities when venturing into new places, which is great, but make sure that you don't slip back into bad habits. Prior to your trip, do a special Visualization Exercise (page 52) that focuses on remaining vape free the entire time. Book nonsmoking, nonvaping rooms. Distract yourself by staying busy as much as possible. Go sightseeing, exercise, and participate in group activities.

Again, you can't control what others around you are doing, but you can avoid situations that will trigger you, and you can and should ask friends and family not to vape around you. If they persist, they're not respecting your best interests, so avoid them to the extent that you can until the cravings no longer tempt you.

Day 15 Assignment

❏ Continue with H2M (page 73) and keep on your NRT (page 55) no matter what.
❏ In your Quit Kit (page 159), identify your most likely social triggers and what action steps you can take to avoid them.
❏ Do your Visualization Exercise (page 52).

Teen Talk: Peer Pressure

Teens have a social trigger that most adults don't. They can feel peer pressure on many fronts, but it's largely internal. They see their friends engaging in certain activities, such as vaping, and they feel an internalized need to join in.

When I was a teen, most of my friends didn't smoke. As I grew older, some of them picked up the habit, and then I did, too. Whenever I was trying to quit, I gravitated toward nonsmoking friends, but when I was smoking, I preferred the company of other smokers because they didn't gripe about the smell or what I was doing to my health.

A 2014 study of two thousand teenagers conducted by the University of Southern California shed important light on the topic. Researchers wanted to learn what most influenced teens to vape. Ultimately they found that young people were more likely to vape if their friends and family approved of it. So peer pressure turned out to play a key role in their decision. The study also revealed that teens are more accepting of vaping than smoking. They know that smoking is dangerous, and even at a young age, they recognize the stigma around cigarettes. But teens rarely condemn their friends for vaping or admit that it's harmful.

If your child has friends who vape, you need to have an honest, nonjudgmental conversation with your kid about those friends, using the principles outlined in "Dear Parents" (Rebel with a Cause, page 37). Remain loving and supportive, and remember that your teen makes lots of smart decisions every day. Resisting the temptation to vape can be one of them. Praise his or her good judgment and encourage positive, independent thinking and principles.

Day 16

Meditate Your Quit

Close your eyes. Relax your body. Breathe. That's all that meditation is. It doesn't have to feel complicated or weird at all.

Meditation is a form of mindfulness that helps you kick nicotine in a number of ways. It naturally and beneficially activates a dopamine pathway in your brain in the same way that an addictive drug, such as nicotine, does. It helps you curb urges by distracting your mind, giving you a new way to relax and manage stress without vaping. Deep breathing also helps make your lungs stronger.

Several studies conducted over the past decade investigated the benefits of meditation to kick the nicotine habit, all with positive results. In one study, published in *Tobacco & Nicotine Research* in 2016, researchers randomly assigned forty-four adult smokers either to a meditation group or to a control group that did primarily breathing exercises. Both groups could smoke as much or as little as they wanted. The meditation group followed a guided meditation for twenty minutes every day for two weeks. At the end of the study, only the meditators experienced a reduction in cravings and cigarette use. The study didn't state the average drop in cigarettes smoked daily but noted that it was significant.

You can meditate in lots of different ways. Try one of these.

Breathing Meditation: Sit quietly, close your eyes, relax, and breathe deeply and slowly.

Faith-Based Prayer: Repeat a religious prayer in your mind, selections from the book of Psalms (*Tehillim* in Hebrew), the five daily prayers in Islam (Fajr, Zuhr, Asr, Maghrib, Isha), or the Metta Prayer or Golden Chain Prayer in Buddhism will do. Try one on, then another, and see what suits you.

Transcendental Meditation: To promote a state of relaxed awareness, mentally repeat a mantra for twenty minutes. Many studies have found that this method of meditation proves most beneficial for people with anxiety.

Muscle Relaxation: While lying flat on your back, slowly tense and relax each muscle group, starting with your toes and working your way gradually to the top of your head.

Guided Meditation: This method usually features a soothing voice that leads you through certain mental scenes to help free you from the grip of your own thoughts. Guided meditations are great for people who have a hard time with other forms of meditation because the voice itself keeps you focused on the meditation.

Moving Meditation: For active or restless people, meditation can feel intimidating, but even if you're running around, just sixty seconds of closing your eyes and repeating one of your calming mantras counts as meditation. Think the phrase, hold it in your mind, and slowly repeat it. That's it. Easy!

Meditation is a simple process, and once you figure out what works best for you, it becomes a great tool in your quitting arsenal.

Day 16 Assignment

❑ Continue with H2M (page 73) and NRT (page 55) no matter what.

❑ Meditate today for at least five minutes and incorporate your Visualization Exercise (page 52).

❑ As you go about your day, practice Meditation on the Move at least three times.

Teen Talk: Guided Meditation

After age nine, children have an awareness of their own thoughts, so teenagers definitely can benefit from meditation, too. Many adolescents suffer from attention disorders, though, so I recommend short guided meditations for them. Play a prerecorded, calming script that takes them through a meditation exercise. YouTube has lots of them, and you can involve your teen in the process by letting him or her select the video. Do the guided meditation along with your child.

Day 17

Stretch Your Quit

For some people, meditation doesn't quite get the job done, and that's OK. Those who require a little more stimulation to focus should stretch themselves—literally. Yoga combines physical, mental, and spiritual disciplines. Using body postures, breathing, and meditation techniques, yoga calms the mind and soothes the body. It improves flexibility, mobility, and strength. It acts as a mood elevator and promotes a sense of well-being. It also gives practitioners a sense of connection to the universe. Think of it as a handy cross between exercise (Day 11) and meditation (Day 16).

From an addiction standpoint, it brings together many of the elements necessary to deal with withdrawal and cravings: cleansing exercise, positive conditioning, and stress relief. It honors and unites body, mind, and spirit in healthy, life-giving ways, and practicing yoga provides a foundation and tools for building good habits. Yoga's effect on GABA, a calming neurotransmitter in the brain, may explain why the practice proves so effective at helping break addictions. Yoga raises GABA levels, which reduce stress and anxiety, both triggers for addictive behavior.

Many addiction specialists use yoga as a therapy for nicotine addicts because it calms the mind, defuses triggers, and strengthens the lungs. It works fast, too. In a study published in *Nicotine & Tobacco Research* in 2018, researchers recruited fifty-five smokers who wanted to reduce their nicotine intake or quit smoking altogether. They randomized them into groups that received one session of yoga or, the control group, that read educational materials about a healthy lifestyle on their Quit Day. The investigators found that just thirty minutes of hatha yoga produced a greater reduction in cravings than the control group that read. If a single session of yoga can work that well, imagine what it can do for you several times a week.

The practice of yoga has formats for all interests and skill levels. Here's a brief overview of the most popular versions.

Yin: Poses, mainly lying down or seated, last for three to five minutes. The longer stretches release tension and restore range of motion to muscles and connective tissue.

Hatha: This format employs sequences of poses and breathing techniques to create calm. The poses change slowly, but holding them sometimes can prove physically demanding. Hatha has become the most common form of yoga practiced in the world.

Vinyasa: Also called a flow class, this variation synchronizes movement with breath as you move from one pose to another in set arrangements. Expect to move faster than in hatha.

Ashtanga: This fast-paced, physically demanding sequence of poses practiced in the same order strongly emphasizes breathing correctly.

Carrie started vaping while in college. "Breaks between classes were my social time. I'd leave the classroom building, go outside, and vape with my friends. But eventually I developed a hacking cough and had a hard time getting up in the morning for class.

"A friend invited me to a yoga class. I was initially resistant," she, a preacher's kid like me, admitted. "I thought it was mostly a religious activity but decided to try it anyway."

Carrie discovered that the deep breathing and breath control exercises helped strengthen her lungs. Yoga also helped her with her anxiety, cravings, and stress. She started going regularly to yoga classes, and a few weeks later she stopping vaping for good.

In the yoga universe, there's something for everyone. Many dedicated yoga studios have beginner classes and workshops that teach the fundamentals. Their offerings work well for first-timers and more advanced students alike. Find a local class that sounds good and fits your schedule. In addition to studios, check out what classes your workplace, gym, or athletic club offers. Not ready to pose in public? No problem. Stream a yoga program or watch one on TV or a DVD and follow along. Also take a look at online options, such as Glo .com, I love teacher Marc Holzman's sessions featured there. If the spiritual aspect of yoga doesn't feel right, then follow a simple posing or stretching routine.

Whichever version you choose, this powerful therapy can help you move through your addiction to become a committed ex-vaper.

Day 17 Assignment

❏ Continue with H2M (page 73) and NRT (page 55) no matter what.

❏ Start by watching a few simple yoga or stretching videos online, then sign up for a class.

❏ Do your Visualization Exercise (page 52).

Teen Talk: Yoga for Teens

Lots of young people do yoga these days, which is great. Yoga has so much to offer them. It teaches teens to cope with anxiety, body-image issues, stress, and uncertainty about the future. Yoga also can help prevent and reduce substance abuse in young adults.

One study, published in 2017 in the *Journal of Youth and Adolescence*, looked at whether the practice could promote smoking cessation in teens. Researchers randomly assigned seventh-grade public school students by classroom either to receive thirty-two weekly sessions of yoga instead of their regular physical education classes or, the control group, to continue with PE class as usual. At the end of the study, the kids in the control group were significantly more willing to try cigarettes than the kids who did yoga, which suggests that school-based yoga can help teens kick nicotine.

Teens can feel awkward trying new activities with their parents, though, so if that's the case, encourage your kid to try yoga with a trusted friend first.

Day 18

Neutralize Negative Beliefs

Developed over a lifetime, your negative beliefs derive from and build on your doubts (Day 6), your emotions (Day 9), and your internal dialogue (Day 12). These beliefs drive coping behaviors or mechanisms that help you manage everything from getting through a bad mood to navigating severe personal trauma.

We rarely admit it—either aloud or even to ourselves—but many of us lug around toxic beliefs about how we relate to others, such as:

1. *I want everyone to like me.*
2. *I need to avoid conflict at all costs.*
3. *If I show who I really am, people will shun me.*

Some negative beliefs focus on capabilities or characteristics. People struggling with addiction often feel innately bad or unworthy, which of course isn't true. You might have made poor decisions in the past or done things that you regret, but that doesn't make you inherently worthless. Downplaying past achievements, strengths, and talents cripples your ability to move forward in life and becomes an act of self-sabotage. If this sounds like you, you may also suffer from low self-esteem, find it hard to love others, and feel pessimistic about life in general. Negative capability beliefs offer lots of "I can't" excuses, which reinforce self-destructive messaging in your brain. If you tell yourself repeatedly that you can't do something, eventually you *won't* be able to do it.

Other negative beliefs make excuses either for us or our behavior. Addicts commonly use everyday situations—arguing with a partner; gaining weight; having a bad day; missing a valuable opportunity; not getting a job, promotion, or raise; or wasting money—as an occasion to abuse alcohol, overeat, vape, or make other unhealthy choices. But here's the thing. Those situations themselves don't cause you to drink, eat, or vape. Your *reactions* to those situations do, and those reactions stem from your beliefs about yourself. If you don't think that you can resist the temptation to vape, then you're not going to be able to do it.

Here are examples of three negative beliefs that specifically apply to vaping and how you can recast them as positives.

1. *I always go back to vaping even when I try to stop.*
2. *I can't quit.*
3. *I never had any bad side effects, so vaping really isn't that bad.*

1. *If I can stop for a few days, I can stay quit for longer.*
2. *I can quit because I don't vape anymore.*
3. *I'm lucky that I haven't had any bad side effects yet, but lots of other people have, so I need to stop before that happens to me.*

Negative beliefs are a choice. You can choose to swallow them, wallow in them, or let them overtake you—or you can choose to neutralize them. Let's deactivate them now.

Day 18 Assignment

❑ Continue with H2M (page 73) and keep on your NRT (page 55) no matter what.

❏ In your Quit Kit (page 159), take away the power of your negative beliefs by recasting them into positive statements.

❏ Do your Visualization Exercise (page 52).

Teen Talk: Validation

Adolescents often are their own worst enemies, and trying to have an honest, rational conversation about a sensitive subject probably results in a lot of blank stares, defensive responses, eye rolling, or stony silence. Teenagers can prove notoriously uncommunicative with their parents because they don't believe that their parents understand what they're experiencing or because they believe that they'll freak out about something.

A good tool to use in those cases is validation. Listen actively and pay attention. Make eye contact, stay interested, and focus on what you're hearing rather than how you want to respond. Calmly recognize and accept your teen's feelings, ideas, or opinions. This validation does *not* mean that you agree with or approve of unhealthy behavior or habits. It just means that you acknowledge that your child has his or her own thoughts or feelings—that's it.

When you do speak, use "I feel" statements. For example: "I feel frustrated when you roll your eyes because I feel like you're not taking what I'm saying seriously." It's harder for them to argue with how you feel. Plus, it helps them understand that their negative beliefs are impacting you negatively as well.

Sometimes your teenager will try to shut you down: "I know, *I know*. Ugh, we've talked about this before!" Hang in there and remain lovingly persistent. This isn't a onetime conversation. Keep the lines of communication open.

Day 19

In Case of Relapse

Staying quit from week to week can predict the likelihood of long-term abstinence. Success generally improves as the number of your vape-free days increases.

But fighting a nicotine addiction is a process—not a one-shot deal. You might lapse or slip and take a drag from someone else's pen. You might relapse after a while and return to vaping regularly. For most people, quitting is a journey, and journeys have uncertainties, challenges, and changes. Wrong turns happen, but they don't mean the end of the road, and they don't mean that you've failed.

Cravings have a real-time life expectancy of about five to ten minutes. They can feel much longer, but really, that's it. If you do slip, your chances of success at getting back on track increase if you have an action plan in place. Even better? You already have every tool that you need for your action plan.

Before we itemize what's in that tool kit, let's look at some of life's red-flag situations and why lapses actually have some benefits.

Bad Cravings: Urges are a normal part of the quitting process, and early on they come from physical withdrawal. Cravings related to emotional and social dependence often arise later. But over time they all become easier to manage.

High-Stress Situations: You know they're coming, but you can't control them. These situations include a divorce, financial worries, getting married, moving, and work deadlines.

Negative Moods: Emotions, as distinct from situations or

events that can cause them, also can cause you to slip—for example: anxiety, depression, and low self-esteem.

Alcohol Use: Drinking impairs your judgment and lowers your inhibitions. You may be more likely to think that just one puff will be OK when it's not.

Social Conflicts: Seeing other vapers might tempt you, especially if they're part of your social group. Arguments or conflict with a spouse or partner, kids, coworkers, or friends might trigger you as well.

Hard Shocks: These you don't see coming, which can make them harder to handle than life's regular stresses. Possibilities include a breakup or divorce, a car accident, the sudden death of a loved one, a diagnosis of a serious illness, or losing a job. When these difficult occasions arise, it's common for people to revert to old coping mechanisms. Vaping might feel like a reward for surviving the trauma, but where's the logic in abandoning your goals and harming yourself as a reward? You're really just punishing yourself.

What if you give in to an urge and vape during this program? A slip or lapse is common. Don't beat yourself up about it and, more important, don't use it as an excuse to quit the program. Instead, use the lapse as a teaching tool for yourself so it can guide you in the future. You can learn and make corrections, to grow in self-awareness by:

- Examining your desire to quit and making a stronger commitment to it.
- Identifying the places, people, or situations you may need to avoid.
- Strengthening your coping mechanisms, such as visualization, H2M, meditation, or yoga.

- Reaching out to your Quit Team for additional help.
- Meeting with your health-care provider to adjust your NRT dosage.

Day 19 Assignment

❏ Continue with H2M (page 73) and keep on your NRT (page 55) no matter what.

❏ Fill out your Relapse Prevention Plan (page 184) and use it as a road map to help you avoid slips.

❏ If you do slip, fill out your Lapse Report (page 184) to keep yourself accountable and focused.

❏ Do your Visualization Exercise (page 52).

Teen Talk: Getting Your Child Back on Track

Above all, stay calm and encouraging. What your kid needs after a slip is assurance and guidance. Remember, he or she might be feeling a lot of guilt and shame that might not be showing. Yelling and throwing your hands in the air aren't going to make the situation any better or help your kid move forward.

Explain that relapse is sometimes a part of recovery. Acknowledge that it's OK to hit a speed bump or to start over. Remind your child of the courage it took to make it this far. Congratulate him or her for progress made and build on that.

Day 20

Health Checkup

At some point during your quit, you probably lamented that you were giving up something you enjoyed, and—let's be honest—you probably felt a little sorry for yourself. But you haven't given up anything except an addiction to poison and a burden on your lungs. You're regaining your physical health. Let's take a closer look at how.

Beyond Withdrawal: In the twenty-four hours following your last vape, you probably had some hard withdrawal symptoms, such as headaches, mood swings, anxiety, or irritability. The worst of it has passed, and you feel better.

No More Vape Nicotine: Three days after you stopped, your body purged all of the vape nicotine from your system, and you felt even less addicted. Cravings still occur, but they come more from habit, and you can handle them better now, including with medical nicotine from NRT

Improved Breathing: Your lungs and airways are working better now, and you can feel it. The inflammation of your lung tissue has lessened, and you're getting more oxygen. You don't experience the same random shortness of breath, you have more energy, and you can do regular daily tasks with ease again, such as walking up a flight of stairs. If you had vaper's cough or an endless cold, it's gone or almost gone now because your lungs can clear themselves and fight off infections better.

Smell and Taste: Vaping dulls your senses of smell and taste. If you love food, the gain here is huge because food tastes good again!

Better Circulation: Nicotine decreases overall blood flow, but your circulation has returned to normal, which results in more physical energy.

A Healthier Brain: Researchers from the University of California, Riverside, have found that e-cigarettes damage neural stem cells, which are as critical as they sound. Nicotine overloads them with calcium, and eventually they rupture.

Reduced Risk of EVALI: Along with measurable improvements in the health of your lungs and heart, this is one of the major health gains of quitting vaping.

Decreased Risk of Heart Attack: If you stop vaping, you'll protect your heart health. A study published in *Toxicology in Vitro* in 2019 found that some chemicals used in e-cig flavorings mess with the heart's ability to pump blood. Researchers at the University of Louisville tested cinnamaldehyde, a common cinnamon flavoring found in vape juice, on the cells in your heart that make it contract. When heated and unheated, the chemical affected the cells' ability to function, and the effect lasted for twenty-four hours. Cinnamon is perfectly safe to eat, but if breathing it can stop your heart from beating, why risk it?

Less Danger of Stroke: Vapers also have an increased risk for stroke, which occurs when something blocks blood from reaching your brain. Quitting decreases this risk almost immediately.

Chance of Cancer Diminishes: We don't know the long-term health effects of vaping yet, but we do know that as soon as you stop inhaling all of those toxic chemicals in vape juice, your risk for all sorts of cancers, including of the mouth, throat, lung, and pancreas, starts to decrease. Quitting gives your body a break!

Day 20 Assignment

❏ Continue with H2M (page 73) and your NRT (page 55) no matter what.

❏ In your Quit Kit (page 159), note how you're feeling better physically. Pay particular attention to the first half of the list above.

❏ Meditate, stretch, or do yoga for five minutes and incorporate your Visualization Exercise (page 52).

Teen Talk: Celebrating Gains

Adolescent bodies are changing constantly, so your child might not notice health gains right away. Make his or her favorite dish for dinner, go through the first half of the health list above, and ask whether and how each one has changed. Praise every improvement.

Day 21

Reward Yourself

You made it to the end of your third week. Congrats! Your body is grateful. Let's take your amazing progress a step further. It's time to reward yourself for all of your hard work.

Rewards incentivize positive behaviors. By replacing the biological or mental gratification of consuming nicotine with a reward, you can keep addiction at bay and reach new milestones.

When you started your quit journey, you probably missed vaping, even though you knew that it was harming your health. Since then, your brain has been going through a lot of changes as it adapts to your new normal. One of those changes is a relative lack of dopamine, a natural feel-good chemical. Rewarding yourself engages the normal dopamine pathway and reinforces it not to want nicotine. In other words, the science says: Treat yourself!

One of the best rewards is a financial incentive. Studies show that monetary rewards help treat addictions very effectively. The larger the incentive, the more effective it is.

Published in *The New England Journal of Medicine*, one trial studied smokers from fifty-four companies. Researchers assigned them to one of four interventions or usual care (access to information on the benefits of quitting and a motivational texting service). The interventions included usual care plus one of the following: (1) free quitting aids (NRT or other medication, with e-cigarettes if standard therapies failed); (2) free e-cigarettes without requiring smokers to try anything else; (3) free quitting aids plus six hundred dollars in rewards for sustained abstinence; or (4) free quitting aids plus six hundred dollar in funds deposited in a separate account for each participant. For group four, researchers removed the money from the account if a participant failed to stay quit for six months after the quit day, and they confirmed whether participants were smoking through urine tests. People in groups three and four had the best quit rates.

Consider making a deal with your spouse, partner, parent, or other close family member or friend who wants you to quit. If you make it to three weeks or a month without vaping, they give you an agreeable amount of cash. Maybe you can make a pool of it with your Quit Team. Everyone throws money into an account, gift card, or pot. If you hit your reward date without vaping, it all goes to you. Save it, invest it, or spend it on yourself.

Rewards can take many different forms, including benefits, clothes, gifts, privileges, trips—anything that you want badly enough to kick nicotine. Here are some easy options for the three-week mark.

- Have your favorite meal at your favorite restaurant.
- Book a massage.
- Hire a babysitter and go on a date night with your spouse or partner.
- Buy a new outfit.
- Go on a gift-card shopping spree.
- Plan a weekend getaway to a favorite spot or somewhere that you've always wanted to visit.

Day 21 Assignment

❏ Continue with H2M (page 73) and NRT (page 55) with medical nicotine.
❏ In your Quit Kit (page 159), brainstorm as many reward ideas as you can to treat yourself for making it this far.
❏ Do your Visualization Exercise (page 52).

Teen Talk: The Cost of Quitting

Vaping isn't cheap, especially for teenagers. Costs vary, but they can run to more than a thousand dollars a year, depending on the equipment and accessories. In five years, that's five thousand dollars; in ten years, ten thousand dollars. Help them do the math and then decide together what happens with all that money: a car, clothes, college, travel, video games, etc. Remember, rewarding them for not vaping rewires their brains, so it's less about where the money goes or what it buys than their enjoyment of whatever that is.

STEP FOUR
STAY STRONG

Days 22–28

I n a boat on the sea, a little boy, just six years old, kept casting his line, trying to catch a fish—any fish. One time, three times, five times, nothing. He started to think that he couldn't do it, but he cast his line a sixth time—and the line pulled back!

All by himself, he struggled to reel in the fish. He pulled and reeled, reeled and pulled. Eventually he hauled a thirty-pound cod, almost as big as he was, from the depths of the sea onto the deck of his father's boat. The boy couldn't believe he had caught such a massive creature. He knew that he had done something special.

"You can catch anything you want as long as you put the effort into it," his father said.

The boy took that lesson to heart as he helped clean the fish. That night, the work of his little hands fed his entire family, and the boy took enormous pride in what he had done—not the least of which was feeding his poor family for several days.

That little boy was me.

What if you changed your mind about what's possible and then achieved it? You can. You, too, can hook the Big Fish and pull a miracle into your boat.

In this step, you will:

- Reset your mind.
- Reclaim your lost time.
- Taper your nicotine intake to nothing.
- Love yourself whole again.
- Connect with a higher power.
- Give back.
- Celebrate your quit.

Day 22

Reset Your Mind

Imagine living in a house with three-foot-tall doors. To get around, you have to crouch or crawl from room to room. Crawling becomes an automatic behavior as you go about your day. You don't even think about it; it's just how you move through the house. When you decide to go to another room, you automatically crouch. This is an example of a mental equivalent, which is an automatic vision, thought, or feeling about something. In our heads, mental equivalents act as templates for how we view and experience the world.

Think the word *door*, and an automatic idea comes to mind of what a door is, how it looks, what it does. You might imagine your front door, the door of your childhood home, a car door, or some other variety. The same goes for any other word, idea, or desire that we have. We all have mental equivalents for our health, relationships, careers, finances— everything. Most of these mental templates work for us. But sometimes, in one area of our lives or another, they need adjusting.

While addicted to vaping, a low mental equivalent deceives you and causes problems in your life. It might convince you that you don't have the power or strength to change. It might make you think that you don't deserve vibrant, healthy lungs and a long, happy life. It sets a low bar for personal achievement and success.

Modeling behavior isn't just something that kids do. It can serve as a powerful tool for personal change by altering unhealthy mental equivalents. Years ago, when I worked as a weather anchor, I was suffering from multiple damaging addictions. Most of my coworkers weren't struggling with similar problems, though, and they seemed happy and well adjusted. The misery of my situation made me want to quit badly, so I quietly studied the people around me, observing their behaviors and how they moved through the world. It didn't occur to me then, but that activity was creating a new mental equivalent for me: a new vision or thought about how nonaddicts act, behave, and live. Doing that helped create a new blueprint for how to live a recovering life. It reset my mental template.

On Day 2, you began to envision yourself as an ex-vaper. In the daily assignments, you've been using the Visualization Exercise to reset your mental equivalent from being a vaper to becoming an ex-vaper. That exercise has been raising the height of the doors in your mental house a little bit more every day.

When you started the program, you probably had trouble envisioning yourself as someone who didn't vape. The Visualization Exercise probably seemed a little weird at first and felt like you were daydreaming about someone else's life. Now you realize you're becoming that person. When you think of yourself now, you don't automatically see yourself as a vaper anymore, right?

Let's build on that progress in today's assignment. Today you're going to become an amateur anthropologist and observe what nonvapers do, how they act and behave. Then you're going to model that behavior and, in the process, reset your mental equivalent. The next time you want to reach for a vape, you'll know how to act like an ex-vaper.

Day 22 Assignment

❏ Continue with H2M (page 73) and medical nicotine in NRT (page 55).

❏ Nonvapers don't hold vape pens in their hands or drag on the devices. So what do they do with their hands? What do they do with their mouths? In your Quit Kit (page 159), observe nonvapers and note the activities that can help you keep your hands busy and what you can do with your mouth instead of vaping.

❏ Talk with at least two people who don't vape and ask them about their daily activities, especially the times when and places where cravings hit you the hardest. Record their answers and your observations in your Quit Kit. If you're not sure whom to ask, tap people on your Quit Team and treat the exercise like an interview.

Teen Talk: Minimizing

Adolescents are pros at minimizing—viewing something as less important or dangerous than it really is—or dismissing things altogether. When deployed to excess, this twisted thinking becomes a kind of psychological junk food. If someone minimizes a real problem, he or she is diluting its seriousness and allowing it to become worse. Users often minimize to protect and prolong their addictions. Have you heard your teen say something like:

"Whatever, it's better/safer than smoking cigarettes."

"It doesn't hurt, so there's no harm in it."

"I'm not addicted. I can stop anytime."

Minimizing blocks recovery, but as a parent you can help smash it. Start by asking your teen gently: "Can you prove that you're not addicted?" Make factual but inclusive counterstatements that disprove any minimization that follows. For example: "We've seen from your latest report card that your grades are falling. We know that you're missing practice, coughing all day, and getting sick more often. You don't think any of that is serious or harmful?"

Then couch your request carefully. Say, for example, "It would make me feel better if I could see that you're not vaping. How about you quit for a week and we see how things go?" A successful trial period will help ease the problem and may inspire a strong-willed teen to take the initiative to quit solo. An unsuccessful trial may prove that he or she needs more intense help. In that case, suggest trying the program in this book.

Either way, as your child starts to quit, emphasize all positive changes. Every few days, ask your child to note the benefits of quitting in terms of breathing, energy levels, money, and so on. Make sure to contrast current gains with past negatives. All of these approaches actively counter minimization.

Day 23

The Power of Time

Not vaping puts time back in your life now and in the long run.

A smoker usually can finish a cigarette in about five minutes. After disposing of the butt, a seriously addicted or stressed smoker might fish a new one from the pack and then light up again. A chain smoker uses the last of the burning ash from one cigarette to light the end of a new one. Each cigarette still takes about five minutes to smoke.

One of the many troubles with vaping is that you can puff continually until the device's battery dies or the pod or cartridge runs out, a behavior called chain-vaping. Case in point: Gerald (not his real name) started vaping in order to give up cigarettes. As is usually the case, his nicotine addiction intensified. He was sneaking drags morning, noon, and night. He neglected his duties at work, frequently missing deadlines, and his duties at home, causing friction with his wife. He developed a chain-vaping habit and was spending hours doing it each day. Gerald was vaping more than he was living, and it was interfering with his relationships, job, and overall quality of life. Vaping controlled him. "Dude, you chain-vape!" his best friend hollered at him.

Any addiction can take over your entire life, as it did Gerald's. You'll use rather than work, study, exercise, pursue a hobby, spend time with friends and family, and other meaningful or productive activities. You lose control of your ability to make healthy choices, and you might find yourself turning to other addictive substances. That loss of control can feel terrifying.

Now that you've reached Day 23, you no longer rely on a vape to get you going first thing in the morning or to keep you going throughout the day. You've regained control of your life in ways and hopefully reclaimed all that extra time that used to go up in a cloud. You feel more present in your day-to-day life. To get to this point, you created your Activity List (page 167). You selected new or more Self-Care Activities (page 83). You changed your routines (page 86). You undertook new or more forms of exercise (page 90). You also made a point to pursue your passions (page 99).

Breaking free from vaping means having a lot more time on your hands, and now you're going to choose how you want to spend that time.

Day 23 Assignment

❏ Continue with H2M (page 73) and keep using medical nicotine in NRT (page 55).
❏ In your Quit Kit (page 159), think of how you want to spend the time that you've reclaimed, both right now and in the future. Look over your Activity List, Self-Care Activities, new routines, exercise activities, and passions list. What do you want to keep doing? What's not on any of those lists that you still want to do or spend more time doing?

Teen Talk: Wasting Time

Even at their best, kids love wasting time. But add vaping to the picture, and they can fall seriously behind in schoolwork or practicing an instrument, language, or sport. The same rules apply to preventing them from wasting time on vaping as on any other disruptive activity, such as excessive use of their smartphone, social media, or video games. First, manage the kid's expectations. Make it clear that changes are coming. Be reasonable, specific, and calm about what you no longer will do or tolerate. Set firm rules, such as no vaping at home, in the car, or at school, and clear consequences. This step in particular gives you more control over the situation, and it also sets clear boundaries for your teen, which all kids need.

Balance any negatives with positives. Point out how much more time your teen will have to do favorite pursuits. Continue to support sincere efforts to quit. Encourage healthy activities in place of vaping. Listen rather than criticize. If you have trouble listening openly and calmly, offer to enlist the help of a school-based support group, counselor, or doctor. This is time well spent.

Day 24

Taper to Nothing

When trying to undo an addiction, a quit curve applies, and it's different for everyone. Some folks quit once, and *bam*— that's it, one and done. Others try quitting again and again, struggling to stop and struggling to stay stopped.

When using medical nicotine in NRT and following the instructions, you've greatly increased your odds of success. It helped weather the toughest physical symptoms of withdrawal from nicotine. By opting for NRT on Day 3, you should have reached your goal of complete abstinence by the third week. That's now!

You've tapered downward with daily NRT use and will discontinue treatment shortly. If you feel that you need NRT for a longer period of time than just the detox part, talk to your health-care provider. To date, studies show negative impact from long-term medical nicotine use. Either way, you're in the homestretch and ready to leap into a vape-free life.

Day 24 Assignment

❏ Continue with H2M (page 73) and use medical nicotine (page 55) as necessary.

❏ In your Quit Kit (page 159), track your NRT progress. How well did it work for you?

❏ Plan a reward for yourself for when you take your final dose.

Teen Talk: A New Attitude

If your kids have made it this far without vaping, that's fantastic. Now it's time to have a new type of discussion. Ask what they think about vaping now. The answers might surprise you. At Breathe Life Healing Centers, we've heard some great insights from ex-vaping teens:

> "I don't want to vape ever again."
> "I heard kids have died from vaping."
> "It's doing some really bad stuff to people."
> "It's incredibly addictive."
> "It's just not cool anymore."

If someone offers them a drag, discuss what to do now. Encourage them to say: "No, thanks. I'm an ex-vaper. I don't vape anymore." Help them see this statement as a declaration of independence. After all, they've broken their dependence on Big Tobacco, which wasn't easy. Praise your child's new attitude.

Day 25

Love Yourself

The greatest power we have in creating change is making people feel loved, yet we use this tool the least. Psychiatrist Karl Menninger put it another way: "Love cures people, both the ones who give it and the ones who receive it."

Love enhances self-esteem and self-worth by helping others see and know their strengths. Love focuses on what's present rather than what's missing. Love offers more joy than material possessions. Love is how much we give of ourselves, how much we share with others, and ultimately how we measure our lives. Nothing else breathes life into us like love. Which explains why a lot of people who don't have it in their lives experience more anxiety, drink more, abuse nicotine, eat junk food, and engage in other self-harming behaviors. I love love!

One of the biggest changes that you need to make for your quit to work is increasing the love that you have for yourself. Lack of self-love can lead to mindless, unhealthy behaviors that trigger addiction and dependency.

A lot of how we view ourselves derives from how we feel about our bodies. It's easy to compare ourselves to people on a variety of screens (movies, TV, social media) or in magazines. But remember that for each of them, a huge team of artists and technicians—personal trainers, hair stylists, makeup artists, wardrobe supervisors, lighting designers, digital retouchers, and more—is turning genetically gifted and incredibly hardworking people into the superhumans we see on screen, stage, and page.

Push those advertising images aside and consider these truths:

- No one else can do things exactly how you do.
- No one else knows everything that you do.
- You are unique in this world.

Learning to love yourself whole again won't happen in a day. For some people, it takes a lifetime. Here's how.

Forgive Yourself: First, go easy on yourself. No one has led a completely blameless or entirely triumphant life. Nobody. So stop beating yourself up for what you've done or haven't done. You can't be happy or free if you continue to blame yourself for events in the past or something that never happened.

Celebrate Wins: The flip side of forgiving yourself is celebrating accomplishments, big and small. Think about all of your successes: showing up, graduating, buying an apartment or house, paying off a credit card or loan, starting a business, cleaning out the garage, learning how to dance, getting married, becoming a parent, beating a personal fitness record, losing or gaining weight.

Mirror, Mirror: Stand in front of a mirror, look yourself in the eye, and say, "I love you. I really love you." It might feel silly, but so did the Visualization Exercise at first, right? As you stand there, think about how you demonstrate your love to your spouse, partner, child, or parent, and imagine loving yourself in the same way.

Personal Promo: What are your talents and gifts? What do you do better than most people? You don't need to be the best in the world or even in the country, but you *are* great at something, and you need to remember that. If you're not sure, ask a loved one for some suggestions. Sometimes other people can see us better than we can see ourselves.

Feel-Good File: Whenever you receive a social media post, letter, email, or text that encourages you and makes you feel good about yourself, save it in a Feel-Good File that you keep in a special place. When you're feeling low, looking through the file will lift your spirits.

Practicing even just one of these simple solutions daily can help you love yourself more. Over time, you'll see big changes in your attitude, behavior, and happiness.

Day 25 Assignment

❑ Continue with H2M (page 73) and medical nicotine (page 55) as is useful.

❑ Look back at your doubts (Day 6) and your internal messaging (Day 12) and see what still feels hard to overcome. Those are the areas where you need to love yourself most. In your Quit Kit (page 159), forgive yourself for those lingering tough spots.

❑ Now that you've forgiven yourself, turn the coin over and note the successes in your life. Use the list above as a guideline and think about what else you've done that makes you feel proud.

❑ Do the Mirror, Mirror exercise. Stand in front of a mirror, look yourself in the eye, and say, "I love you. I really love you." Think about how you show your love to the most important people in your life. How can you love yourself in the same way?

❑ Start your Feel-Good File (page 194). Keep filling it with any messages of encouragement that you receive. When you feel down and need a boost, take the time to read through them.

Teen Talk: The Power of Love

Being a teen these days can feel harder than it ever did before. In addition to authority figures, their peers, and the regular media urging them to achieve more, be better, and look better, kids now feel added pressure from social media platforms. For example: not racking up the same number of followers or likes as their friends, or feeling excluded when seeing classmates and friends having fun without them. All of which can cause teens to suffer from a lack of self-love.

You can help your kids recognize their worth, reclaim their self-love, and pursue a healthy and positive future. Try the following activity with your kids or encourage them to do it on their own. All your teen has to do is fill in the blanks.

- My teachers say I'm really good at:
- My friends like to hang out with me because:
- Three qualities that I like about myself are:
- I'm really proud of:

It's not easy to up a teen's self-love game, but you can encourage and celebrate abilities, skills, and talents so that they feel more inspired, confident, and capable—now and for the rest of their lives.

Day 26

Connect with a Higher Power

Many addiction programs exclude spiritual practice from the treatment process, often against the desires of patients and to their detriment. Not everyone is religious or spiritual, but those who are need that element in recovery programs. Spirituality is highly personal.

Studies by the National Institute for Health Research (NIHR) show that participation in religious worship can help ease stress, lower blood pressure, alleviate symptoms of mental illness, prevent addiction, and even help protect against cancer. The NIHR has found that prayer and religious commitment can improve recovery rates and shorten the length of hospital stays as well. No doubt the social setting and support structure play a key role in those findings. If you're suffering and need help, people in a faith-based community reach out and help. A North Carolina study found that frequent churchgoers had larger social networks with more contact with, more affection for, and more support from their religious communities than unchurched people.

One size doesn't fit all. Some people don't believe in organized religion but do feel a sense of personal spirituality. Others don't believe in spirituality but acknowledge the existence of an unknowable higher power. Still others don't believe in any kind of supreme entity at all. All of which is totally cool. Whether you practice a particular religion or are a spiritualist, agnostic, or atheist, most will benefit from an awareness of what fulfills us on a higher level. When you find that, you can make it an identifiable piece of your life that provides solace, energy, and hope.

You don't have to be religious or spiritual to engage in or benefit from prayer, either. It's just a form of intention setting, kind of like programming a destination into an internal GPS that serves as a focal point for your consciousness. That intention gives you a direction and destination.

At their most basic level, all forms of prayer are saying: "Hi, it's me here, I'd love to connect. I'm having trouble, and I need help." That's it. When you seek connection with God, the universe, friends, or family, you're setting an intention for what you want to happen. Remember the Law of Attraction from Day 2 (page 51)? Prayer calls that law into action.

You can repeat an established religious prayer that gives you comfort and strength. The Serenity Prayer is a great, easy option. ("God, grant me the serenity to accept what I cannot change, the courage to change what I can, and the wisdom to know the difference.") You can unite yourself with an abstract notion of the divine or mystical. You can write your own prayer, commune with nature, engage the fellowship of friends, or connect with the beauty showcased in your favorite museum, symphony, or song. However you do it, the act of asking for help has real power.

Determine your intention and embody it in short, positive phrases or sentences that express where you want to focus your attention and energy. Then let go of your pride and your ego and ask for help. This is my daily prayer, which has changed over the years, as I practice it today:

"To the spirit of life, I offer myself. To build and lead and do with me as is right. Guide me in letting go of pride and ego, that I might do what I am meant to do. Help me deflect

roadblocks of fear, that victory in tough times might demonstrate how truth and good and love, if allowed, guide me."

Day 26 Assignment

❏ Continue with H2M (page 73) and NRT (page 55) as much
as is useful.

❏ If you're having trouble with your quit, harness the
intention-setting power of your preferred method of prayer
today. Use the space in your Quit Kit (page 159) to help
focus your thoughts and write your own prayer.

Teen Talk: Courage, Serenity, and Wisdom

When they're younger, kids come to parents when they need
help, which, at its most basic, is a kind of prayer. You're the first
line of support for your kids when they're dealing with bullying,
friends, school, and other stresses. When they're struggling, you
want them to feel comfortable turning to you.

When your kids are in trouble or need help, let them know
you're always available, unselfishly and with love. If your teens
come to you with a problem, tell them you're proud of them for
sharing it with you. Voice your appreciation of the courage that
it took to ask for help. Respond positively and give them your
full attention. Then share a brief story of a similar problem that
you or a close friend or family member had. Discuss how you or
the other person asked for help and ultimately resolved the
problem. As with adults, sometimes teens just need an ear to
listen or a shoulder to lean on. Ask if they want to know what
you think they should do. Offer your advice only if they say yes.

What if you don't have all the answers? That's OK. As a parent or guardian, it's fine to admit that you don't know everything. But if your child asks for help, make every effort to offer support or find someone, such as a coach, counselor, doctor, or psychologist, who can. You may not always be able to intervene, either. Your teen may need to work it out solo or seek help from another authority figure. Sometimes, as the Serenity Prayer tells us, you need the courage to know when to help your kids, the serenity to know when to hold back, and the wisdom to know the difference.

Day 27

Give Back

"I can't quit!" because "I have quit!"

As you look back on your quit journey, think of all the people who helped you do it. In incredible ways, an act of service—helping another without pay or recognition—empowers us. Service connects us to those in need, reminds us of when we also needed help (to quit, to grow, to thrive), and puts our own needs in perspective.

If you don't do it already, it's time to extend a helping hand. Some people call it paying it forward, but you don't have to spend any money to do it. You just need to find a way to give meaningfully to someone who needs help. An obvious place to start is to mentor or sponsor someone struggling with vaping, but the options are endless. Consider participating in one or more of the following activities.

- Become a school crossing guard.
- Collect school supplies for special-needs classrooms.
- Create care packages with essential items.
- Donate blankets to a homeless shelter.
- Donate blood.
- Donate food or your time to a soup kitchen or food bank.
- Help adults learn to read.
- Knit socks for the homeless.
- Organize a clothing drive.
- Pick up garbage at a local park or beach.
- Rake leaves or shovel snow for someone who can't.

- Read to kids at a public library.
- Register as an organ or tissue donor.
- Request charitable donations instead of birthday or holiday gifts.
- Visit with or read to seniors at an assisted-living facility.
- Volunteer at an animal shelter.
- Volunteer at a women's or youth shelter.

If you do, you'll find that you get a lot in return. Your self-esteem will swell, and you'll feel both helpful and useful. When you bring a little joy into someone else's life, joy will come into your own as well.

Day 27 Assignment

❏ Continue with H2M (page 73) and NRT (page 55) as much as is useful.
❏ In your Quit Kit (page 159), note how others have helped you on your journey to stop vaping. How are you paying it forward or giving back to them or others?

Teen Talk: Giving Back

Again, the obvious place for your kid to start is to mentor or sponsor another child struggling with vaping. The Preventing Tobacco Addiction Foundation posted a great story on their website (tobacco21.org) about an example at Orange High School in Ohio.

A senior at the school tried to quit vaping several times, but his failure made him feel hopeless. He consulted the school psychologist, who gave him some strategies. The sessions helped, and the senior successfully quit vaping. He wanted to give other students that same opportunity, so he shared the strategies with one friend, then another. Soon he formed a peer support group.

Now kids as young as age fifteen who want to quit vaping attend a weekly gathering where they share their successes and setbacks. No administrators, no teachers, no parents. With teens, peer-to-peer help is *much* more effective than hearing from parents or other adults. See if your kid's school has such a group or if someone wants to start one.

A lot of schools have community service requirements for graduation, which unfortunately can make giving back feel like a chore or yet another task to complete. If your teen is struggling with ideas, steer him or her toward possibilities that align with existing hobbies or passions. What skills does your child have that can help others?

Day 28

Celebrate Your Quit

You never thought you'd be able to quit vaping, and here you are—successful! As different as you've become from the vaper you were a month ago, imagine how different you'll be in a year. Imagine how your lungs are honoring your good work with each breath! Congratulations!

You made it this far. Now commit to never go back.

Why? You need to *stay* quit or else risk falling back into a vape-y pothole again. Reintroducing a drug to one who was once addicted reignites the chemical dependence fire. Unfortunately, it happens all the time. That's why those "in recovery" say that they're in recovery for the rest of their lives. They know how quitting and staying quit are the journey of a lifetime. If you vape again—yes, even just *one* drag—regardless of how in control you feel, it can suck you back in, and you'll have to go through the whole process all over again.

Some people have harder, longer quit journeys, and they relapse. If that happens to you, chin up! Remember that people who love and respect themselves don't abandon their goals and punish themselves in the guise of a "reward." Life's hard shocks (page 121) are tough, but they're not worth the costs of living as a vaper again.

As of today, you officially have completed your quit. In medical terms, you are now in recovery from a vaping addiction. You've done much more than that. You've refined who you are and how you want to live your life. You've become an ex-vaper. Wear the badge of success loudly and proudly.

Tell your story to others. Continue to share your journey with your Quit Team and others. Join our Facebook group to join your tribe!

Start by celebrating the new you with them by hosting a Quit Party. Invite your Quit Team and other friends and loved ones to a tobacco-free gathering at your home, a restaurant, a public park, or any place that feels comfortable and inviting. Cook for it, have it catered, or have everyone bring something. Share your story and thank your team, person by person, for helping you on your journey. Then ask them to share their positive stories about your journey and messages of encouragement.

With each day that you spend as an ex-vaper, the odds increase that you will stay stopped for good. You now have the power to move forward, you know which choices to make, and you understand how you want to breathe through the rest of your beautiful life.

Day 28 Assignment

❑ Read your Quit Kit (page 159) all the way through, from start to finish. Note the feelings, discoveries, and other insights it contains. Revisit how you managed doubts and triggers. See how your routines and emotions have changed, giving you the confidence and determination that you need to live your life vape free.

❑ Fill out your Certificate of Achievement (page 197).

❑ Take a picture of your Certificate of Achievement and share it, along with a selfie of the brand-new you, with loved ones and on social media.

❑ Host your Quit Party. Remember, this is a big deal, so make sure that everyone knows it!

Teen Talk: The Dead-Man Rule

When dealing with your kids, always try to follow the Dead-Man Rule. Never ask them to do something a dead person can do. Only dead people cannot act or not behave a certain way. Instead, rephrase your directives positively.

Consider a typical scenario: Your teen repeatedly leaves his or her dirty clothes on the bedroom floor. If you repeatedly shout "Don't leave your clothes on the floor!" your child repeatedly hears a negative. When kids continually hear negatives, the words lose their impact, and your kiddo will tune you out, as you might have experienced already. Better to say: "As soon as you take them off, put your dirty clothes in the hamper or laundry basket." Emphasize the behavior you want to encourage, and you'll get better results.

When it comes to vaping, flip negative commands—"Don't you dare start vaping again!" or "Don't even think about taking another puff!"—into what they should do instead, such as: "If you feel the urge to vape again, let me know, and we'll check in with your support group" or "Read through your Quit Kit if you feel like you need help." Empower your teens to do what they should do rather than forbid them to do what they shouldn't.

Part Three

Your Quit Kit

QUIT CALENDAR

Day 1
Your Quit Day:
___/___/___

Day 2
**Envision Becoming an
Ex-Vaper**

Day 3
Replace and Taper

Day 4
Nutritional Detox

Day 5
Assemble Your Quit Team

Day 6
Defeat Your Doubts

Day 7
**Practice H2M and
Begin NRT**

Day 8
Clean House

Day 9
Emotional Cues

Day 10
Change Your Routine

Day 11
Exercise Your Quit

Day 12
Monitor Your Messaging

Day 13
Recognize Your Progress

Day 14
Pursue Your Passions

Day 15
Social Triggers

QUIT KIT

This Quit Kit provides valuable tools and exercises that will reinforce your resolve to stop vaping. It can help when you're struggling, and it will also give you perspective on how far you've come when you read back through it.

On the pages that follow, you'll find day-by-day support for dealing with cravings and handling triggers, and lots of prompts that will propel you on your journey. This tool kit contains a number of questions that ask you to explore your feelings, emotions, and behaviors to keep you on the path to becoming nicotine free. Answering them honestly will enable you to tackle the challenges that come your way and face them successfully.

Change requires both determination and action, so decide to act now. Follow the program in this book, do your daily assignments, and use the Quit Kit to discover the path to your new vape-free life.

Day 1
Your Quit Date Promise

Rewrite the following text onto the lines below, then sign and date your promise. Take a picture of it, and share it with loved ones and on social media—including to our Quit Vaping support group on Facebook!

> On [date], six days from today, I will quit vaping. I will repeat this commitment the next day and the next, conquering one craving at a time, until I am an ex-vaper!

_____

_____

_____

Signature: _____

Date: ____/____/____

Day 2
Envision Becoming an Ex-Vaper

How will your life look when you quit? Think about what
will be different after you quit and describe those changes
below.

_____

_____

_____

_____

_____

_____

_____

_____

_____

_____

_____

_____

_____

_____

_____

_____

_____

_____

Commitment Quiz

Which myths about vaping resonated with you and why?

_____

_____

_____

Are you addicted to nicotine? _____

How does that make you feel?

_____

_____

Do you know anyone who has had health problems
because of vaping? What were they?

_____

_____

_____

If your lungs could talk, what would they tell you?

_____

_____

_____

How will your life improve after you quit?

_____

_____

_____

As a percentage, how committed are you to your quit right now?

_____ %

Vision Board

Let's be creative in this! Gather your supplies. You'll need scissors, glue, and the board itself, which can be a simple sheet of paper or something bigger and sturdier.

Find a good, joyful picture of yourself from before you started vaping and print it out in color.

Flip through your favorite magazines or newspapers and tear out any images or words that appeal to you. Scroll through your favorite social media accounts and also print out in color any images or words that make you feel good about your future. These could be happy photos of loved ones, images of activities you want to do, pictures of places that you want to visit, quotes that inspire you, or anything that represents a happy, vape-free life. Trust your intuition. You'll know when it feels right.

Glue your photo to the center of your Vision Board. Then arrange the inspiring images and words around it and glue those down as well.

Day 3
Replace and Taper

Do your Visualization Exercise (page 52).

Day 4
Nutritional Detox

Do your Visualization Exercise (page 52).

Day 5

Assemble Your Quit Team

Who Is Your Quit Team?

Name at least five people who want you alive and to quit vaping. Might you enlist one of them as your Quit Buddy? If so, who?

_____

_____

_____

What Do You Want to Hear from Your Quit Team?

For example: "I'm so proud of you." "How can I help you kick your habit?" "What else would help you feel better?" What else do you want them to say or ask you? Write more options below.

_____

_____

_____

_____

Escape Plan

If you need to avoid people who tolerate or encourage vaping, how are you going to do that? What are you going to say to them? Write your plan and the script for that sentence below.

_____

_____

_____

_____

Activity List

What activities with family and friends will help you avoid the temptation to vape? List at least five below and then make concrete plans—date, time, place—to do them.

_____

_____

_____

Day 6
Defeat Your Doubts

Which self-doubts resonated with you the most? Do you have others? Write each of them below in red, leaving spaces between each one. Underneath each doubt, rephrase it into a positive truth in your own words in a different color.

_____

_____

_____

_____

_____

_____

_____

Breakup Letter

Which of the doubts above worries you the most? Circle it. Now write a breakup letter to that doubt below. Explain how it hurt you, why it doesn't deserve your time anymore, and why you need to move on. Share this to our Quit Vaping Facebook group to encourage others and yourself.

_____

_____

_____

_____

Day 7

Practice H2M and Begin NRT

More Mental Mantras

Which of the affirmations (page 74) feel best to you? Might others work better? Write them below.

_____

_____

_____

_____

_____

Day 8

Clean House

Clean House Checklists

Here are two checklists to help you ditch any physical reminders of your past vaping life. The first one lists all the places that you might be keeping vaping paraphernalia. Go through each place carefully and toss *everything* that has to do vaping.

- ❏ Backpack
- ❏ Bag
- ❏ Balcony
- ❏ Basement
- ❏ Bathroom
- ❏ Bedroom
- ❏ Bookshelves
- ❏ Car
- ❏ Closets
- ❏ Coats
- ❏ Coffee table
- ❏ Deck
- ❏ Den
- ❏ Desk
- ❏ Dresser
- ❏ Foyer
- ❏ Garage
- ❏ Garden
- ❏ Guest room
- ❏ Jackets
- ❏ Kitchen
- ❏ Liquor cabinet
- ❏ Living room
- ❏ Messenger bag
- ❏ Nightstand
- ❏ Office
- ❏ Pantry
- ❏ Purse
- ❏ Shed
- ❏ Study
- ❏ Yard

Now here's a checklist of the items to chuck. Don't save anything "just in case."

❏ Adapters

❏ Atomizers

❏ Batteries and chargers

❏ Build kits

❏ Coils and cartridges

❏ Drip tips

❏ E-cigarettes

❏ E-liquids

❏ Labware and mixing supplies

❏ Mods

❏ Pods

❏ Replacement glass

❏ Starter kits

❏ Storage bottles

❏ Tanks

❏ Vape pens

❏ Vaper T-shirts or other pieces of clothing

❏ Vaping apps or links on phones, tablets, and computers

❏ Vaping ads, articles, brochures, or other printed material

❏ Wire, wick, and cotton

❏ Any other reminders that you used to vape

Day 9

Emotional Cues

Which three emotions or feelings on page 78 are your most frequent triggers to vape? Identify them below and explain what usually causes each emotion and how vaping helps you cope with them? For each one, what can you do instead of vaping? Trauma survivors are more prone to addiction than others. What past hurt enables self-soothing with vaping?

_____

_____

_____

_____

_____

_____

_____

_____

_____

_____

Emotional Mantras

Using the list of Mental Mantras on page 74, write a couple of short, strong sentences that you can use as mantras to deal with your three vape-triggering emotions above. For example, if you fear that you won't have any friends if you stop vaping, try something like this: "I will overcome this fear and live my new life with courage."

_____

_____

_____

_____

_____

_____

Self-Care Activities

When you're feeling emotional, which Self-Care Activities (page 83) will work best for you? What else might help? Write them below.

_____

_____

_____

_____

Day 10

Change Your Routine

What three routines automatically prompt you to vape?
What are some good habits that can replace them?

_____

_____

_____

_____

_____

_____

Day 11
Exercise Your Quit

What physical activities on page 90 do you enjoy doing most? What are some that you've never done but you want to try? Now's the time! List them below.

_____

_____

_____

_____

_____

What's your fitness goal?

_____

_____

_____

Day 12
Monitor Your Messaging

Internal Dialogue

Is your self-messaging positive or negative? Below, list the
five thoughts that you have most often about yourself. Are
any of them positive? If so, circle them. Now look at the negatives. Rewrite each one as a positive statement and draw a
line through the negative thought above it. So I'll never be
able to stop vaping becomes: With practice and encouragement, I am learning how to quit.

Day 13
Recognize Your Progress

To honor changes you've made and the progress that you're making, answer the following questions in detail below.

How does your body feel? What are your lungs telling you in this moment? When you're not fighting a craving, are your moods better? Do you feel stronger? Do you have more energy? Can you breathe more easily? What might you do better?

_____

_____

_____

_____

_____

_____

_____

How much money have you saved by not vaping for the past two weeks?

$_____ × 26 = $_____ that you'll save in one year. What do you want to do with all that money? Do you want to save or invest it or treat yourself or a loved one? What kind of special reward might you want for the first anniversary of your Quit Day?

_____

_____

_____

_____

What are you doing with the daily time that you don't spend
vaping? Is there anything else that you'd like to be doing?
What do you want to do in the future?

_____

_____

_____

_____

Day 14

Pursue Your Passions

What Are Your Passions?

Answer the following questions in detail below.

What fills you with anticipation?

What can you do over and over and never get bored?

What do you wish you could do all day long?

_____

_____

_____

_____

_____

_____

_____

_____

_____

Day 15
Social Triggers

List your top three social triggers below. They can be people with whom you used to vape, people who still vape around you, or places where you used to vape. What happens or what are you afraid will happen in each case? Do your cravings increase? Do you slip and feel guilty afterward? In each case, what can you do to avoid and prevent these social triggers?

_____

_____

_____

_____

_____

_____

_____

_____

_____

_____

_____

_____

Day 16
Meditate Your Quit

Practice meditation in conjunction with your Visualization Exercise (page 52). Remember, H2M is a moving meditation. You're doing great!

Day 17
Stretch Your Quit

Do your Visualization Exercise (page 52).
   Practice H2M (page 73).

Day 18
Neutralize Negative Beliefs

Following the examples on page 117, fill in the blanks below.

I always _____

I can't _____

I'll never _____

I'm a _____

My relationships suffer because _____

When things go wrong, I _____

Now rewrite each of those negatives into a positive in the space below.

_____

_____

_____

_____

_____

_____

_____

_____

Day 19

In Case of Relapse

Relapse Prevention Plan

What are you afraid will cause you to lapse? See the list on (page 120) for reference and fill in the following table.

Possible trigger	Is it environmental, emotional, behavioral, or social?	Note the corresponding day (8, 9, 10, 15) in the program and review it.	What can you do to prevent it from triggering you?	What will you do if you slip?

Lapse Report

If you do lapse, that's OK, but you need to figure out why so you can prevent it from happening again. If it happens, fill in the following table.

Lapse action	What led to the lapse?	What can you do differently in the future?	What will get you back on track?	What did you learn?

Day 20
Health Checkup

In the space below, write down how your physical well-being has improved. How are your cravings now? How is your breathing? What do your lungs tell you in this moment? How are your energy levels? How do food and drink taste?

_____

_____

_____

_____

_____

_____

_____

_____

_____

Day 21
Reward Yourself

In addition to your favorite options listed on page 127, how else might you treat yourself? Write them all down below and then number them from smallest or cheapest to biggest or most expensive. Now you have a handy list of rewards for future milestones (one month, two months, and so on). Plan to reward your future success.

_____

_____

_____

_____

_____

_____

_____

_____

Day 22
Reset Your Mind

Modeling New Behaviors

Discreetly observe people in public who don't vape. What are they doing with their hands? What are they doing with their mouths? Which of those activities can help you fight the urge to vape? List the activities below.

_____

_____

_____

_____

_____

_____

Talk with at least two people who don't vape and ask them about their daily activities. Focus on the times when and places where cravings hit you the hardest and ask what they do with their hands and mouths. Record their answers and your observations below.

_____

_____

_____

_____

_____

Day 23
The Power of Time

Think about how much free time you have since you stopped vaping. What new activities that you started doing to help quit vaping do you really like? What else sounds appealing? Travel? Trying a new hobby? Spending (more) time with loved ones?

_____

_____

_____

_____

_____

_____

Day 24
Taper to Nothing

NRT Questionnaire

This survey helps draw attention to the progress that you've made by using NRT. Look over the following eight statements and rate how using medical nicotine has worked for you. Indicate your responses as follows: 1 = did not help; 2 = helped moderately; 3 = helped greatly. Be honest.

NRT and the tapering process:

Eased my withdrawal symptoms (cravings, anxiety, depression, sleeplessness, etc.).

  1   2   3

Helped me focus on productive activities other than vaping.

  1   2   3

Made me feel less addicted to nicotine as I tapered.

  1   2   3

Relieved strong emotions or feelings, such as anger and distress, as I tried to quit vaping.

  1   2   3

Was useful in helping me change habits and be more productive.

    1   2   3

Contributed to a greater sense of well-being (more energy, better breathing, mental focus, etc.).

    1   2   3

Increased my motivation to quit as the program progressed.

    1   2   3

Helped me stay stopped.

    1   2   3

Add up the numbers you circled: _____
Now multiply that number by 4: _____

If NRT was a test, that second number reflects the score for how well it worked for you. The highest score is 96, which indicates that NRT worked exceptionally well. If you scored somewhere in the middle, around 64 points, or lower, look back at the statements for which you circled 1 or 2. If the NRT isn't helping, you might need to work on better habit formation, emotion management, or other aspects of your quit. Go back and revisit the days in the program that address these issues.

If you've tapered to nothing, reward yourself with one of the ideas that you listed on page 187.

Day 25

Love Yourself

Forgiveness

Using Day 6 and Day 12 as guides, determine what you might forgive yourself for. How would you have done things differently if you had had the skills or insight that you have now? What did you learn in the process? Why are you grateful for that experience? How will you forgive yourself now?

I forgive myself for

_____

_____

_____

_____

_____

_____

_____

_____

_____

Your Wins

List five meaningful personal successes below. Use the list on page 141 as a starting point but think of some of your own. How did you achieve each win or success? What skills or talents did you apply to make each one happen?

_____

_____

_____

_____

_____

_____

_____

_____

_____

Talents and Skills

List below at least three skills or gifts that you have. Give a couple of recent positive examples of how you used them in your life. Ask your Quit Team to help you with this one.

_____

_____

_____

_____

_____

_____

_____

Feel-Good File

Write "My Feel-Good File" on the tab of a file folder. Print or add any social media posts, letters, emails, or texts of encouragement that you receive. Make sure to include the person's name and the date of the message on the note. Keep the folder in a special place and pull it out when you need to remind yourself how awesome you are.

Day 26

Connect with a Higher Power

The Power of Prayer

Prayer is just a statement of intention. There's no right or wrong way. If you need help getting started, try writing your own prayer below. Join me on our Quit Vaping Facebook group to connect.

Begin with gratitude and acknowledge something for which you're grateful. Then focus on an issue with which you need help: withdrawal symptoms, cravings, a health concern, staying quit, guidance, or something else. What are you struggling with? For example: *I am struggling with _____. I'm afraid it will interfere with my recovery, affect my life, and cause harm. I need help finding the right path forward.*

Day 27
Give Back

How have how others, especially your Quit Team, helped
you along your journey? Share your reflections below.

_____

_____

_____

_____

_____

How can you help others in a similar way?

_____

_____

_____

_____

Day 28
Celebrate Your Quit

Date and print your name on your Certificate of Achievement below.

Certificate of Achievement

FOR QUITTING VAPING

This certifies that on this day, _____ , 20___ ,

_____

[YOUR NAME]

stopped vaping. The above person did it one second,
one minute, one day at a time and pledges
to repeat this commitment tomorrow, the next day,
and the next to stay quit for good.

Appendix

How to Intervene

Working for twenty years as an interventionist with people who need help getting back on track has made me certain that people can change. Sometimes it just takes more in-depth help. Most adults and teens who vape to satisfy a nicotine addiction can quit with the program offered here, but some will find change extremely difficult and uncomfortable or remain reluctant to try. For some, gentle persuasion, encouragement, reasoning, begging, or nagging can't over-come that reluctance. But they aren't hopeless. They might just need to go through an intervention, and some kind of more intensive treatment.

For the reluctant to change, an invitational intervention is a powerful tool. Its purpose is to convince someone that he or she has a serious, perhaps life-threatening problem that requires help. An invitational intervention is a meeting in which you face your loved one and explain that you are concerned about his or her health and well-being. From this starting point, hopefully you can direct the person toward a doctor, detox program, or support group that can help him or her face the realities of suffering and start on the path to recovery before the situation worsens.

More specifically, an invitational intervention provides

an opportunity for loved ones to offer examples of how a problem has proven destructive or detrimental both to the loved one and to those around them. It gives health-care professionals and loved ones the opportunity to explain a course of treatment that they think will work best. It also can showcase for the one suffering the consequences of his or her actions if choosing not to accept further help. Invitational intervention uses only as much pressure as needed, leveraging relationships to help jump-start change.

For the hard to change to make genuine progress, an intervention is a critical option. As a loved one, you're in a perfect position to help your vaper alter his or her act because that bad habit is more than just an annoyance. It has the power to sicken or even to kill. Asking another to seek help can be one of the most important requests that you ever will make.

Plan the Intervention

An invitational intervention requires thought, planning, and attention to your loved one's needs and circumstances. It's a good idea to contact a therapist or counselor for help in planning it. You can invite one or more medical professionals to participate in the intervention so they can provide relevant medical and treatment information. The planning stage consists of four elements and is a family meeting by another name.

First, you decide who will attend the intervention—who cares about your loved one and is willing to help. This step crafts the circle of change. The circle of change generally includes the following voices that matter in the life of your loved one:

- Identified Loved One (ILO)
- Friends and immediate family
- Grandparents, cousins, aunts, uncles, and other extended family
- Teacher, past or present
- Counselor, therapist, or social worker
- Health-care professional, physician, nurse, or pediatrician
- Pastor, priest, rabbi, or other member of the clergy

If the ILO is a child, a parent typically leads the intervention team. If the addict is married or has a partner, the spouse often leads. If the ILO has mental illness or has displayed violent or self-harming behaviors, a professional interventionist should join the circle. Visit our Quit Vaping Facebook group for suggestions on qualified intervention support in your area.

In the second step of the planning process, each person who has agreed to join the circle of change prepares a heartfelt message about why the ILO should quit. These declarations help the addict understand the concerns and feelings that everyone has about his or her health and well-being.

The messages should contain no attacks, nagging, or other verbal sparring. Write the messages in a loving way, using eyewitness and flash-forward language. An eyewitness account offers specific instances during which the addict's behavior became scary, destructive, or out of control. Message on these themes: What have you seen? What are your fears? What is your hope?

Here's an example:

> "John, you have friends who vape every day, and you
> hang out with them a lot. Vaping clearly has become a
> big part of your life. I'm worried about you because I
> see you vaping more than ever. You're coughing, short
> of breath, and not focused on work or fun activities.
> You're not living a happy, productive life anymore."

A flash-forward of your hope paints a clear picture of how
you see the addict's life progressing if the addiction goes
unattended, and what positive change you want to see.

Here's an example:

> "I love you, and I'm afraid you're cutting your future
> short. I want you to stop vaping because we all want
> to have you around for a long time. We will support
> you through the challenging process of quitting and
> choosing life."

Each person in the circle should commit their messages
ahead of time and be ready to express them face-to-face,
heart to heart at the intervention.

Third, decide where to hold the intervention. I always
suggest meeting in comfortable, familiar surroundings, such
as someone's home. Do what you normally would do as a
family or with friends: gather for a meal, eat a pizza together, and so forth.

A few additional ground rules: no phones, no arguing, no
preaching, no bad-mouthing. Everyone should remain focused and keep an honest, loving, dignified tone.

Finally, you need to invite the ILO to attend the meeting. You might phrase it something like this:

> "Tom, because we love you, we're having a meeting at eleven today with your mom, your siblings, your best friend, Aunt Cindy, and Mr. Miller, your gym teacher. We're doing this because we're afraid for you and your health. Your mom and I don't know how to handle the situation, so we've asked for help about how we can help you. We're going to have the meeting with or without you, but it's important to all of us that you join us. We love you so much. We want to talk with you instead of about you."

Hold the Meeting

If you're leading the meeting, open with a calm, warm welcome to everyone and thank them for attending. Next, each member of the team will share his or her message, one by one, using the prepared eyewitness and flash-forward accounts described above. The goal here is for your loved one to see how many friends, relatives, and others are willing to offer support, which may be exactly the boost of encouragement needed to start quitting.

Once every member of the circle has spoken, the intervention leader should present the ILO with detailed suggestions for treatment. This step delivers the invitation to change. Suggestions might include attending an addiction treatment program, setting a quit date, joining a support group, seeing a doctor, signing up for a cessation workshop, and so forth. He or she can accept the invitation then and there, or the team can give the addict a day or two to think about it.

Here's an example:

> "Jeremy, we want you to free yourself from this addiction so that you can live life more productively and fully again. We've come together to support you and recommend a treatment program to help you overcome your nicotine addiction. We want you to enter the program at [institute or recovery center], and we want you to agree to this plan. We will take you there, and we will help you change and heal."

If your loved one agrees, make use of a Change Agreement. The ILO agrees in writing to certain commitments: to quit what ails them, to start therapy, take a workshop, attend a support group, etc. The agreement includes reasonable expectations as well as fair consequences if your loved one breaks the terms of the agreement. It also may state that the ILO agrees to take part in regularly scheduled family meetings, for example. Everyone in the circle of change signs the agreement, and everyone gets a copy of it. Here's an example that you can use with a vaper:

Change Agreement

We all agree that vaping is a severe health hazard, which is why we have come together to demonstrate our love and to help Tommy quit. We, the undersigned, will act as his support system, encouraging his progress and helping him avoid relapses.

Tommy, we want you to do the following without negotiation or delay:

1. I will quit vaping on ____/____/____.
2. I will attend vaping cessation classes at the hospital once a week, on Thursday nights from 7:00 p.m. to 8:30 p.m.
3. I agree to follow the quit-vaping plan as outlined by this group, including changing my lifestyle in positive ways (exercise, healthy nutrition, breathing exercises, meditation, and other tools).
4. If I relapse or abandon the above commitments, I agree to residential treatment to help me stop.

Signatures:

_____   _____

_____   _____

_____   _____

Date: ____/____/____

Attach clear consequences for not following the terms of the agreement. Consequences show how serious the intervention team is and can include use of things like the car or other privileges, or ceasing financial support until he or she is willing to begin getting help.

Make sure the consequences are time limited and task oriented. That means, in the simplest form, that if you take something away, your loved one should know what change needs to happen (no more vaping) in a specified short-term period of time in order to earn back a privilege. Let's say your teenager is still vaping. As a consequence, you will keep their phone until he can go three weeks without vaping. Talk. Teach. Test . . . that is, test their urine or saliva to ensure compliance. During that time, they will work on making the change. If successful, your teen gets their phone back.

Pick only one consequence at a time, though. Multiple consequences can create resentment and block change. Stacking consequences prompts the addict not to care about changing.

Quitting is harder for some people than others. Give room for them to learn healthier behaviors. It takes time to realize that you are all serious about the consequences. Don't get discouraged and give up if the vaping doesn't stop right away. Let the consequences do their work and give them time to sink in. Think about speeding tickets. Just because a driver doesn't slow down after the first ticket doesn't mean the ticket didn't work. It just takes some people longer than others to learn to follow imposed limits.

What if your loved one says no to the invitation to change? In some cases, an ILO isn't self-aware or willing to accept responsibility for the problem. The intervention itself also may trigger additional behavior problems that can complicate relationships between the ILO and the intervention team. If the answer is a hard no, take a break and reconvene in an hour. Repeat the request. Try to motivate again but don't nag. With many people, it takes awhile to absorb the gravity of what people are saying. They have to think it over. Be patient.

No matter the outcome of the intervention, it's important to be patient and stick to your plan. Don't give in and don't give up! Invitational intervention works. Doing so will help the ILO realize the impact that their vaping is having on friends and loved ones and may encourage positive change. The whole purpose of intervention is to help your loved one begin a journey to stop vaping.

Champion the Change

To quit, an addicted loved one must overcome a physical addiction to nicotine as well as a psychological dependence on vaping. Therapies such as NRT—medical nicotine—help with the chemical component, but beating the psychological addiction is the hardest part. For many, vaping relaxes them and has become an integral part of daily life. If that's the case, change the collective routine. Help your loved one avoid situations that might trigger failure. Let's use the example of the morning cup of coffee with a vape. Distract your loved one first thing in the morning or guide him or her to an alternate activity, such as meditation, followed by a cup of tea.

Your ILO may have to avoid certain situations, such as hanging out with friends or joining the weekly poker game. Help identify alternative ways to reduce stress, such as exercise, yoga, gardening, or doing a hobby. Do these activities with your loved one whenever the urge to vape strikes.

Provide psychological encouragement. Many people don't have the motivation to quit because they believe they can't. Offer recurring positive input: "Dude, you're doing great. I'm so proud of you!" Then focus on the positives. Talk about how quitting has helped in terms of better health, money saved, improved appearance, more energy, greater

self-confidence, and so on. Congratulate successes and encourage continued abstinence. Reward progress with something meaningful: cash, a gift card, an expensive dinner, an
outing, or some other present.

You also might get results by saying less and modeling
healthy behavior, such as runs or hikes, yoga, going to the
gym, or meditation. Chances are that your actions will pique
your loved one's interests in a healthier lifestyle. Men and
women of all ages are more likely to develop healthier lifestyle
habits when their family members set positive examples.

If a setback occurs, don't get upset. Remind your loved
one that it's a learning experience and relapse sometimes
happens. You don't want him or her to think of it as a failure. Encourage a reset to get back on the vape-free train.
The misstep was nothing more than getting off at the wrong
station. Urge him or her to get back on, try again, and hang
in there. The cravings will pass, and in time the space between them will increase.

It's perfectly fine to prohibit vaping in and around your
home or presence. Your loved one may not like it, but reducing the opportunities to vape helps people quit. Ultimately,
you can't control the addict's behavior, but you can make it
harder to indulge the addiction.

Care for Yourself

You clearly want your loved one to quit before it's too late.
While that's happening, continue your own healthy lifestyle
and guard your emotional well-being. Spend time on yourself so that you don't lose all your energy. Trust the plan to

do its work. Make a life for yourself that doesn't involve twenty-four-hour policing of the addict's vaping habit. When you practice proper self-care, you put yourself in a better position to support your loved one. Visit our Quit Vaping Facebook group and see what other support from your "village" you might find there!

Acknowledgments

When I started writing about e-cigarettes, it was to understand how the newest addiction craze came to be and how it was being marketed as safe. I wondered how a book one day might shed light on what is at its core an addiction like any other. It seemed likely that corporate greed, not care for the global village, was leading the explosive growth. It seemed like a grand, nefarious drive to profit at the expense of the addicted, those afflicted with and affected by trauma. What damage to the precious lungs across the globe was taking place right in front of us? What damage to our loved ones' pulmonary systems would time reveal?

The manuscript stayed in my backpack for more than two years in various stages of research, writing, and rewriting. "You're gonna finish it soon, I know it," my husband, Scott Sanders, often told me. I love love.

Over the years, many people have helped me achieve more than my due. I will try to remember as many of them as I can here.

Oprah Winfrey, thank you for your friendship and for touching my life. In remarkable ways, your support increased how I have helped others.

Dr. Oz, my friend and teacher, you asked me to join you that first year as your talk show launched. We have helped millions of people live better and longer lives as well as shown them how to help those they love. Thank you again for contributing the foreword to this book.

Maggie Greenwood-Robinson, please accept my heartfelt thanks. You are loyal and brilliant. I am the luckiest guy to get to be your collaborator. Tara Filip, keeper of my keys and coconspirator in bringing my ideas to light, this book would not have found completion without you. Todd Shuster, thanks for being more than an agent; you are a true creative partner. Your team at Aevitas, including Justin Brouckaert and Erica Bauman most of all, are the best in this business.

To Stacy Rader and her team at *The Dr. Oz Show*, thank you for telling stories over the years that I care so much about. I have seen families find help and healing through the stories you have mined and invited in.

Mindy Borman, Julie Cooper, Lisa Erspamer, and Conrad Shadlin, you made me teach better on television than I really am. I have loved every minute of work and play. Tim Sullivan, you have made the messenger incredibly grateful and magnified my ability to teach and tell. Thank you so much.

Terence Noonan and Marc Malkin, you are my friends and playmates in spreading stories that are good times and good-for-the-soul times. Scott Lamm, do you remember the first one?—written into being with your dream that I would and could write that first book so many years ago. I love you, brother. Gregg Lamm, Dad wanted me to tell you that he would come to the wedding all over again if he could. With all of my brimming heart, I am my father's son, a Lamm boy even now.

Deb Hughes, my mentor and teacher more than all but few. Kathleen Murphy, LMFT, LPC, the most skilled healer, you give me the possibility of change even in the most wounded.

Mackenzie Phillips, did you think we'd get so good and lucky in surviving and then thriving? Marvin Schwam, you were my family when it felt like the world was over for me. I feel like the third Schwam boy on some days. Thanks for loving me, Freddy and Matthew. Jeanette Fein, you helped me in finding a path when newly recovering. Owen van Natta, you have helped my "spin cycle" spin in better ways.

James Jayo and Patrick Nolan at Penguin Books, I am grateful for your interest in this book and the good it will do.

Dr. Mike Crupain, I treasure your talents and time spent with me. You've made the stories I have shared on air better, no doubt.

To all those helped by this work, you give me something great in return: purpose.

Notes

Introduction

Barrington-Trimis, J. L., and A. M. Leventhalm. "Adolescents' Use of 'Pod Mod' E-Cigarettes—Urgent Concerns." *The New England Journal of Medicine* 379 (2018): 1099–1102.

Christiani, D. C. "Vaping-Induced Lung Injury." *The New York Times*, September 6, 2019.

Hoffman, J. "Addicted to Vaped Nicotine, Teenagers Have No Clear Path to Quitting." *The New York Times*, December 18, 2018.

Howatt, G. "Minnesota Reports 2nd and 3rd Deaths from Vaping-Related Lung Disease." *Minnesota Star Tribune*, October 16, 2019.

Richtel, M., and D. Grady. "Cases of Vaping-Related Lung Illness Surge, Health Officials Say." *The New York Times*, September 6, 2019; updated October 8, 2019.

Richtel, M., and S. Kaplan. "First Death in a Spate of Vaping Sicknesses Reported by Health Officials." *The New York Times*, August 23, 2019; updated October 8, 2019.

Myths and Truths

Alzahrani, T., et al. "Association Between Electronic Cigarette Use and Myocardial Infarction." *American Journal of Preventive Medicine* 55 (2018): 455–61.

American Association of Poison Control Centers. "E-Cigarettes and Liquid Nicotine." https://aapcc.org/track/ecigarettes-liquid-nicotine.

Boretsky, A., et al. "Nicotine Accelerates Diabetes-Induced Retinal Changes." *Current Eye Research* 40 (2015): 368–77.

Breland, A., et al. "Electronic Cigarettes: What Are They and What Do They Do?" *Annals of the New York Academy of Sciences* 1394 (2018): 5–30.

Butt, Y. M., et al. "Pathology of Vaping-Associated Lung Injury." *The New England Journal of Medicine* 381 (2019): 1780–81.

"Exploding E-Cigarette Kills 24-Year-Old Texas Man." BBC.com. February 5, 2019.

Gaur, S., et al. "Health Effects of Trace Metals in Electronic Cigarette Aerosols: A Systematic Review." *Biological Trace Element Research* 188 (2019): 295–315.

Grady, D. "Lung Damage from Vaping Resembles Chemical Burns, Report Says." *The New York Times*, October 2, 2019; updated November 9, 2019.

Henry, T. S., et al. "Imaging of Vaping-Associated Lung Disease." *The New England Journal of Medicine* 381 (2019): 1486–87.

Kaplan, E., and J. Hoffman. "Juul Knowingly Sold Tainted Nicotine Pods, Former Executive Says." *The New York Times*, October 30, 2019; updated November 20, 2019.

Lauren, F. C., et al. "Pulmonary Toxicity of E-Cigarettes." *American Journal of Physiology—Lung Cellular and Molecular Physiology* 313 (2017): L193-L206.

Lee, H. W., et al. "E-Cigarette Smoke Damages DNA and Reduces Repair Activity in Mouse Lung, Heart, and Bladder as Well as in Human Lung and Bladder Cells." *Proceedings of the National Academy of Sciences of the United States of America* 115 (2018): E1560-E1569.

Martin, E. M., et al. "E-Cigarette Use Results in Suppression of Immune and Inflammatory-Response Genes in Nasal Epithelial Cells Similar to Cigarette Smoke." *American Journal of Physiology* 311 (2016): L134-L144.

Olfert, I. M., et al. "Chronic Exposure to Electronic Cigarettes Results in Impaired Cardiovascular Function in Mice." *Journal of Applied Physiology* 124 (2017): 573–82.

Primack, B. A., et al. "Initiation of Traditional Cigarette Smoking After Electronic Cigarette Use Among Tobacco-Naïve US Young Adults." *American Journal of Medicine* 131 (2018): 443.

Richter, L, "10 Surprising Facts About E-Cigarettes," CenterOnAddiction.org, October 2018.

Roseberg, E. "Exploding Vape Pen Caused Florida Man's Death, Autopsy Says." *The Washington Post*, May 17, 2018.

Rossheim, M. E., et al. "Electronic Cigarette Explosion and Burn Injuries, US Emergency Departments 2015–2017." *Tobacco Control* 28 (2019): 472–74.

Shields, P. G., et al. "A Review of Pulmonary Toxicity of Electronic Cigarettes in the Context of Smoking: A Focus on Inflammation." *Cancer, Epidemiology Biomarkers & Prevention* 26 (2017): 1175–91.

Soneji, S., et al. "Association Between Initial Use of E-Cigarettes and Subsequent Cigarette Smoking Among Adolescents and Young Adults: A Systematic Review and Meta-analysis." *JAMA Pediatrics* 171 (2017): 788–97.

Song, M. A., et al. "Effects of Electronic Cigarette Constituents on the Human Lung: A Pilot Clinical Trial." *Cancer Prevention Research*, October 16, 2019.

Spicuzza, M., and R. Rutledge. "11 Wisconsin Teens and Young Adults Hospitalized with Lung Damage Linked to Vaping, and Seven Other Cases Are Under Investigation." *Milwaukee Journal Sentinel*, August 2, 2019.

Tommasi, S., et al. "Deregulation of Biologically Significant Genes and Associated Molecular Pathways in the Oral Epithelium of Electronic Cigarette Users. *International Journal of Molecular Sciences*, February 10, 2019.

Visser, W. F., et al. "The Health Risks of Electronic Cigarette Use to Bystanders." *International Journal of Environmental Research and Public Health*, April 30, 2019.

Nicotine Addiction

Aleyan, S., et al. "Risky Business: A Longitudinal Study Examining Cigarette Smoking Initiation Among Susceptible and Non-Susceptible E-Cigarette Users in Canada": *BMJ Open* 8 (2018): e021080.

Hughes, J. R., et al. "Withdrawal Symptoms from E-Cigarette Abstinence Among Former Smokers: A Pre-Post Clinical Trial." *Nicotine
& Tobacco Research*, July 28, 2019.

Ibarra, A. B. "Vapers Seek Relief from Nicotine Addiction In—Wait for
It—Cigarettes." *California Healthline*, September 13, 2019.

Wickham, R. J., et al. "Evaluating Oral Flavorant Effects on Nicotine
Self-Administration Behavior and Phasic Dopamine Signaling." *Neuropharmacology* 128 (2018): 33–42.

Dear Parents

Aubrey, A. "She Survived the ICU. Now, She Has a Message: Quit Vaping!" NPR.com, October 9, 2019.

Grady, D. "Facing 'Certain Death,' Teenager with Vaping Injury Gets
Double Lung Transplant." *The New York Times*, November 12, 2019.

Notley, C., et al. "Incentives for Smoking Cessation." *Cochrane Database
of Systemic Reviews*, July 17, 2019.

Step One: Plan Your Quit

Hartmann-Boyce, J., et al. "Nicotine Replacement Therapy Versus Control for Smoking Cessation." *Cochrane Database Systematic Reviews*,
May 31, 2018.

Lindson-Hawley, N., et al. "Gradual Versus Abrupt Smoking Cessation:
A Randomized, Controlled Noninferiority Trial." *Annals of Internal
Medicine* 164 (2016): 585–92.

Patten, C. A. "A Critical Evaluation of Nicotine Replacement Therapy for
Teenage Smokers." *Journal of Child and Adolescent Substance Abuse* 9
(2000): 51–75.

Scaglia, N., et al. "The Relationship Between Omega-3 and Smoking
Habit: A Cross-Sectional Study." *Lipids in Health and Disease*, March
22, 2016.

Step Two: Manage Your Cravings

Conklin, C. A., et al. "Exercise Attenuates Negative Effects of Abstinence During 72 Hours of Smoking Deprivation." *Experimental and Clinical Psychopharmacology* 25 (2017): 265–72.

Faria, L. M. "Portugal Solved Its Drug Crisis. Why Can't America Do the Same?" *Huffington Post*, November 11, 2019.

Step Three: Live Your Quit

Barrington-Trimis, J. L., et al. "The E-Cigarette Social Environment, E-Cigarette Use, and Susceptibility to Cigarette Smoking." *Journal of Adolescent Health* 59 (2016): 75–80.

Butzer, B., et al. "Evaluation of Yoga for Preventing Adolescent Substance Use Risk Factors in a Middle School Setting: A Preliminary Group-Randomized Controlled Trial." *Journal of Youth and Adolescence* 46 (2017): 603–32.

Halpern, S. D. et al. "Randomized Trial of Four Financial-Incentive Programs for Smoking Cessation." *The New England Journal of Medicine* 372 (2015): 2108–17.

Jeffries, E. R., et al. "The Acute Impact of Hatha Yoga on Craving Among Smokers Attempting to Reduce or Quit." *Nicotine & Tobacco Research*, December 14, 2018.

Nystoriak, M. A., et al. "Comparative Effects of Parent and Heated Cinnamaldehyde on the Function of Human iPSC-Derived Cardiac Myocytes." *Toxicology in Vitro*, September 10, 2019.

Ruscio, A. C., et al. "Effect of Brief Mindfulness Practice on Self-Reported Affect, Craving, and Smoking: A Pilot Randomized Controlled Trial Using Ecological Momentary Assessment." *Nicotine & Tobacco Research* 18 (2016): 64–73.

Zahedi, A., et al. "Mitochondrial Stress Response in Neural Stem Cells Exposed to Electronic Cigarettes." *iScience* 16 (2019): 250–69.

Step Four: Stay Strong

Hardison-Moody, A., and W. M. Stallings. "Faith Communities as Health Partners: Examples from the Field." *North Carolina Medical Journal* 73 (2012): 387–88.

Koenig, H. "Religion, Spirituality, and Health: The Research and Clinical Implications." *ISRN Psychiatry*, December 16, 2012.

McIntyre, Michael K. "How Pervasive Is Teen Vaping? Students at This Local High School Formed an Addiction Support Group." *Cleveland Plain Dealer*, February 3, 2019; updated February 5, 2019.

Resources

Various organizations offer great resources for quitting vaping. Here's a selection of them.

American Cancer Society
250 Williams Street NW
Atlanta, GA 30303
(800) 227-2345
Cancer.org

American Lung Association
55 West Wacker Drive, Suite 1150
Chicago, IL 60601
(800) LUNG-USA (586-4872)
info@lung.org
Lung.org

Breathe Life Healing Centers
8730 Sunset Boulevard, Suite 550
West Hollywood, CA 90069
(888) 765-0610
BreatheLifeHealingCenters.com

**Centers for Disease Control
and Prevention**
1600 Clifton Road, MS E-90
Atlanta, GA 30333
(800) 232-4636
CDC.gov

**Campaign for Tobacco-Free
Kids**
1400 I Street NW, Suite 1200
Washington, DC 20005
(202) 296-5469
info@tobaccofreekids.org

**Parents Against Vaping
e-cigarettes**
ParentsAgainstVaping.org

Tobacco 21
youth@tobacco21.org
Tobacco21.org

Truth Initiative
900 G Street, NW, Floor 4
Washington, DC 20001
(202) 454-5555
TheTruth.com
TruthInitiative.org